REVIEWS OF THE DIGITAL EDITION

"So much variety. It will take a while to try them on. When you find one you like, you want to keep making it over and over. So much wonderful information and wonderfully delicious recipes. Well worth buying this!" – Lorraine

"Love this collection of recipes from Amanda Rose. There are so many delicious recipes to try. Easy and nutritious, anyone can whip these up. You have to try the pizza in a bowl or Reuben in a bowl, my favorites. Not just recipes but a strategy for 'good days' and not so 'good days'. What to eat, when, and how, lots of good information here." – Linda

"I have been an Eat Like a Bear member for over a year and have lost 55 lbs. so far. I love the Ridiculously Big Salads from Amanda's other book, but now I have even more choices. I can never say that this way of eating is boring or has no variety and these recipes aren't diet food, but real delicious meals that are just healthy." – Eva

"This isn't your run of the mill 'diet cookbook'! If you're looking for amazing, easy, healthy recipes to help you lose weight, you wouldn't be wrong. My favorites: Zuppa Toscana Soup, Chicken Salsa Verde and the Pizza Skillet. But wait . . . this book is so much more! Amanda and her team have given you a framework to craft and create meals on your own. They have given you strategies to help with your health journey, which makes the purchase price the best investment you can make for your health." – Debie

"Another fabulous addition to the RBS library! So many great meals to help us stay focused on days we need something warm! The framework and the process is simple and has proven results! What a great value and worth every penny! Thank you, Amanda!" – Georgia

"As a seasoned cook and chronic dieter, this WOE is changing my life. I love the simplicity of the ingredients and instructions, plus they help me make use of the proteins and veggies I get in my weekly farm box without the need to spend hours in the kitchen 'creating' dishes. Thank you, Amanda Rose, for investing your heart and time into something that is changing lives forever." – Linda

"Got it. Recipes are terrific! Love the shopping list for the week! Easy to do. I have to do all the cooking for my ailing wife, so easy is great!" – William

"I already have the RBS Half My Size hardcover book and truly appreciate that all of that 'stinkin' thinkin' which that vindictive little demon on my shoulder whispers in my ear can be diverted away from just by directing my attention to Dr. Rose's RBS recipes as I peruse them the evening before and make my decision as to which one to choose for my meal the next day. And now I proudly own her latest addition and am thrilled to see a myriad of yummy hot meal recipes to choose from as well as I continue to successfully grind. Brilliant, Dr. Rose and thank you for such top quality, motivating books and mentorship!! Hugs from Florida!" – Lani

"I grew up with a dog-eared copy of Peg Bracken's *The I Hate to Cook Book* on our kitchen shelf; its formulaic recipes let my cooking-resistant mother pass dinner prep on to her 5 daughters. In *Half My Size with Soups, Skillets, and Sautés*, Amanda Rose sets you up for success by making ELAB's one ridiculously big meal a day so easy you could do it in your sleep if you had to; she knows from personal experience that on some days that's all that we can manage. For possibly food-addicted folks who struggle with their weight (probably not uncommon in the ELAB community), this easy to master formula for food prep gets us cooking, but thankfully for such a short and simplified time, the demons around preparing and eating food are held at bay. And while she stresses multiple times that these recipes are not geared towards winning culinary awards, I've found them to be the type of delicious and satisfying comfort food I usually associate with carb-laden dishes. As someone in maintenance (yay, ELAB!), I also like the rigor of the formula, which makes it easy to rein in and correct the 'poundage creep' that sometimes comes with increased eating flexibility. It's a long term and extremely manageable strategy that teaches you how to think as much as what to cook."

"Thanks Amanda Rose, for providing a format that can take me into a healthy and EASY future with food. Great book; great recipes. Bring on the hardcover edition. I'm sure it will be dog-eared in no time!" — Bebe

"Got it, Read it, Love it!! If you're looking for more out of the RBS and ELAB or just love the Cooked RBS recipes, then don't hesitate . . . not only does it pack great recipes but you get a WHOLE LOT more! I love the recipes, but the psychological aspect of this book is top of my list!!" — Sue

"I am so so so happy to have this publication/way forward to ELAB! The psychological info and the description/approach to the recipes are so clear and helpful. I am retooling my mind/heart and ACTIONS to ELAB with hot/cooked foods MOST EVERY DAY! God bless you and your team, Amanda!!!!" — Wendy

"Love this! The KISS (keep it simple sweetheart) method works especially well on your good days and days you might struggle on. There's a framework that makes it easy to apply to every recipe. I read it all the way through my first day. Read the all the chapters, in order to best succeed! Thanks Amanda!" — Jude

HALF MY SIZE WITH THE

Ridiculously BIG Skillet

AMANDA ROSE, PH.D.

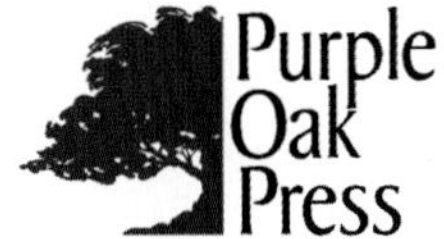

Published by Purple Oak Press

Book Design by Peter Holm,
Sterling Hill Productions

Cover photo by Jen Williams,
Willis and Williams Design Studios

Printed in China through
Porter Print Group, Bethesda, MD

ISBN 978-1-934712-22-1

First Printing

MEDICAL DISCLAIMER

The content in this book is not intended to be a substitute for professional medical advice, treatment, or diagnosis. For all medical conditions, concerns, or questions, always seek the advice of your physician or other qualified health or medical services provider. Do not disregard professional medical advice or delay in seeking medical care or advice based on the contents of this book or any ancillary materials or communications by its author.

contents

chapter one

The Origin of the RBS Framework

I am not sure of the common path to writing weight loss books, but my own path seems fairly backward, and so I will attempt a brief introduction.

I lost 140 pounds (64 kilograms) in just over a year in 2017 and 2018 in a process that I never imagined would work. I certainly never imagined I would end up at my lowest adult weight and start the Eat Like a Bear! community, with tens of thousands of people adopting the same approach and losing life-changing amounts of weight as well.

Here I am now, writing a book about a very specific and distinct way of eating, and the odd part is that, as I went through my own weight loss phase, I had no real appreciation for the distinctiveness and replicability of my meal approach. I was just working something out for myself. The food was low in carbohydrates and calorie minded. I ate it all in one meal.

When people started asking about it, that is simply what I taught: ratchet down your carbohydrates and rein in your eating time.

We had thousands of people doing just that, working out their own food plan with those general instructions. We had a community culture of eating diversity, within the general framework of reducing carbohydrates and paying attention to eating times. In those early community days, I just kept on eating my own giant salads and skillets as others ate whatever they chose to eat.

It would be nearly a year before community members prodded me into the kitchen to measure everything I was eating. The community was asking for a book about salads, a project I could not imagine was worth anyone's time and surely would have no interest.

As I replicated my weight loss meals in that kitchen one year after my own weight loss phase, I was shocked to discover how absolutely consistent my weight loss meals had been. Even though my own brain created them, I had not appreciated how systematic they were. These meals were a serious monument to my technocratic side.

Then something even crazier happened: I released that early salad book, an early version of *Half My Size with the Ridiculously Big Salad,* and we saw the success rate in the community go up as a result. The community itself essentially taught me the effectiveness of this way of eating, with massive amounts of social proof.

Have you ever made a bunch of big changes, had great results, but then were never really sure which of those changes were actually important? That was me in 2018.

Yes, I had great personal success, but it was the community success with this eating framework that helped me learn how effective my specific eating model was. In that year before my realization, I was eating other keto foods and playing around with various maintenance strategies, many times verging far from my main meal framework. I wonder if I would have ended up far astray without the community. In fact, I do often wonder if I would have gained the weight back without the role of the community in providing me with social proof of this particular meal type.

This book is all about the Ridiculously Big Skillet. It's the cooked version of the popular meal framework at Eat Like a Bear! called the RBS after its predecessor, the Ridiculously Big Salad.

We call it the RBS these days, but this meal framework mirrors what I ate to lose 140 pounds (64 kilograms) over the course of about a year. In my early rapid weight loss days, I ate the salad version of this meal probably about every four out of five days. I varied my eating with a cooked version of the meal. As the RBS framework has grown in popularity as a result of the success of *Half My Size with the Ridiculously Big Salad,* I've been asked for nearly two years to write a spin-off book about that fifth day of my eating. This is that book.

ITERATING MY WAY TO THE RBS SOLUTION

In the fall of 2017, I was deep in my head "iterating" my way through finding my optimal meal type for weight loss. When statisticians talk about iteration, they are referring to the mathematical process of optimizing an outcome; it entails repeating a process until the best possible outcome is achieved given the available data. For decades I had never considered using this research approach to my weight loss problem. As a trained statistician, I suppose it was natural for me to approach my eating challenges from this viewpoint, but I simply had never done so before.

As it was, I went through this process of iteration out of desperation. I was scheduled to have bariatric surgery in four months and was determined to walk into that surgery with no regrets, having done everything I could on my own to lose weight. I found myself in a unique psychological position, and without consciously intending to, I launched into a mindset that would change my life.

To iterate my way to an optimal diet, I imagined the whole landscape of food choices available: all the fast foods and their various options (from the fries to the lettuce wraps), all the many combinations of things we might eat at home, all the many diets from Mediterranean to paleo to keto. I used my decades of experience in weight loss attempts to inform my choices.

My first choice in the process was to eat nothing, and I went on an extended fast in the very beginning. As I lay on my couch eating nothing, knowing that eating nothing was not actually a sustainable decision, I began to make choices in that landscape of tens of thousands of options. I knew that certain choices would not take me where I needed to go, and so I could ignore the options of french fries and donuts and zero in on some options that might yield success.

From my many other diets, I knew that low-carb eating was effective, and I knew that calories mattered. I had heard a lot of reviews about time-restricted eating, and so I decided to combine these three approaches and eat one low-carb, calorie-minded meal in one hour. I had struggled with hunger on all of my past diets, and so I selected a meal that had bulky items that would fill me up but would not be high in calories. I wanted to make sure I felt stuffed so that I could get through until the next day.

I began by eating a giant salad every day. Over some weeks, I continued to eat a giant salad for the most part, but I refined the meal itself, adapting it to my daily experience. I did two key things: I increased the daily calories a bit, and I implemented cooked versions of these salad meals that followed a similar framework.

It took weeks of implementation for me to land on this eating framework. It is a process I worked through on a day-to-day basis, iterating toward the best solution for myself. I altered the specifics of my eating choices, depending on the feedback I received from my own experience. Not full enough? Eat more greens! Concerned about enough calories? Add more calories! Tired of a raw salad? Cook the vegetables!

It's a strange thing that it took me forty years to approach my eating problem like a scientist, but that's exactly what happened in the fall of 2017—but not like a scientist who has to prove anything to other scientists or who is attempting to prove or disprove a scientific theory. I wasn't trying to create a framework that would stand up to the rigors of peer-review research.

I had an audience of one: me.

I had to prove to myself that I had done everything I could do to lose weight, and so I made choices iteratively responding to all of my own self-doubt and second-guesses and landed on an optimal meal type in the process.

In retrospect, it's likely a good thing I had no idea that my process would end up with a curious audience of tens of thousands of people. In fact, I was so mentally focused on this mindset of "proving to myself before bariatric surgery" that I iterated for more than two months before I realized that the process was so successful I would not need bariatric surgery after all.

I had salads more often than these skillet and soup dishes because I found the salads to be more satisfying, and I was less likely to get as hungry as quickly. Simply, the Ridiculously Big Salad is a better tool for me for the long haul, from a satisfaction and hunger point of view.

However, the cooked version of the meal framework did provide me with variety, which became an important tool for that long game of weight loss. And there are a good number of people who can't eat salads for various digestive reasons, in which case the cooked version of the framework is exactly the place to start.

It is the cooked versions of those meals from that fall of 2017 that are in this book.

This book also shines a light on the structures in your life that have caused you to pack on those pounds. Change those structures, and those changes will help you not only lose the weight but keep it off. I write this having beaten all odds against maintaining my own 140-pound weight loss after a lifetime of maintenance failure. I leaned hard into this psychology content in the fall of 2021 when my family was evacuated in the Windy Fire, a wildfire that ravaged the Sequoia National Forest, killing dozens of thousand-year-old giant sequoia trees and coming within a mile of our property on three sides. Nothing tests your pant size like losing your entire lifestyle in one fiery weekend.

What makes both the RBS and the cooked version successful is not the ingredients or cooking method but the mindset. If you can understand a bit about why the framework is driving success apart from the specific recipe ingredients, it will help you to adapt it better to fit your needs and to meet your long-term goals.

Draw the Line and Walk Away

The Eat Like a Bear! community has had massive weight loss success with this meal framework, but is it because I have somehow landed on the exact list of ingredients we have all been searching for our entire lives? Does this book contain a specific ingredient list that is the sole solution for weight loss?

For those familiar with this framework and the Eat Like a Bear! community, you already know my answer: no.

From the point of view of its specific food content, the RBS framework is not really revolutionary. There are many weight loss approaches that dance right around this RBS method, using similar food choices, and yet the success rate of people following the RBS framework is far higher than those following other similar models. If our eating is nearly the same, what else are we doing that drives our higher success rate?

Despite our impressive success, not everyone in the Eat Like a Bear! community who has implemented the framework is meeting their goals. We also have people bouncing around in their weight. Why is that?

The answer is: choosing the right food to eat is necessary, but that alone is not sufficient. *How* you use the framework to change your life may be the important point in all of this.

Eating the RBS or something similar may be a required component for successful weight loss (as may those variations that dance all around it), but it may not be enough in itself. That is to say, you may need to implement the RBS framework along with some other elements to have both the necessary *and* sufficient conditions for weight loss and weight maintenance.

My own implementation of the RBS framework all those months had the necessary conditions of a calorie-minded, carbohydrate-restricted satiating meal that reduced my body's insulin resistance, but it also allowed me to leverage one of my very best psychological tools (one that I am well known for among friends and family, for better or for worse): I can purposefully "forget" about something, and I do so regularly. Your psychologist would call it disassociation. We all do it to some degree or other, some of us better and more consciously than others. It can get us into all kinds of trouble if we "forget" important things because we mentally shoved them aside.

If you've found me here at a higher starting weight (as many people do), you are likely as skilled at forgetting as I am. Do you know how I know? You cannot survive in our modern culture, fat, without some strategic disassociating. If you've survived the shame and judgment to get you to the point of reading this book, you have likely used this very strategy. Shame over being fat is pervasive in our culture, and it lives deeply in many of us.

But in the case of daily eating, we can most definitely use this powerful skill. Take your pro skill at forgetting and ignoring your shame and turn it into the most productive tool in your tool belt. Use it in a proactive manner to build the life you want to live.

Our entire culture is structured to keep us thinking about food, and that is exactly why we are all so fat. What if we purposefully ignored all those cultural signals that got us here? What if you enjoy one giant satisfying meal each day, take in that satisfaction for a few minutes, and then "forget" about food for the next twenty-three hours? That is essentially what I am suggesting.

Eat strategically during a specific portion of the day, and if you need to be extra-intensive with your weight management, eat the meal within one hour. Enjoy that meal, but make it calorie- and carb-minded like the RBS. Be satisfied and then forget about food.

Yes, I am well aware that hunger will creep up later in the day and that you are going to want to eat during those other hours. I am also well aware that if you give in and cross that boundary, the overall effort to stick with the framework and lose weight gets much more difficult. The fight to keep eight almonds from becoming two cups, day after day, is far worse than drawing the line and not eating those eight nuts in the first place.

And that mindset is how I achieved my weight loss of more than 100 pounds (45 kilograms). For many months, I ate my one meal each day and then I walked away from food.

I recommend that approach to people all the time: "Draw the line and walk away!" I have said it often, but people hear it in different ways, and it is my purpose to shine a bright light on that point in this book.

THE RBS FRAMEWORK AND THE GOOD DAY STRATEGIES

Some years ago, I wrote a book called *Rebuild from Depression: A Nutrient Guide* and also sent out an email newsletter on depression. The book centered on depression and food nutrients, and the newsletter focused on what I called "Good Day Strategies." I'm going to give you a classic example of a Good Day Strategy for depression and argue that the RBS framework may be the ultimate in Good Day Strategies for fat loss and weight maintenance.

In the context of depression, I argued that to get us through those dark days, we should work on our good days to establish structures for our mental health, structures that would still be there on bad days and could make those bad days a little less bad.

A classic example of this from my own life begins with a large stand of lemon balm I planted one day in the summer of 2012. As lemon balm is a hardy perennial that spreads easily, I could have just tossed a few seeds on the ground and waited a year. But I was feeling good that summer and apparently wanted a project, so I rescued lemon balm from various areas of our property where the seedlings would have needed to be pulled anyway, planted them in pots, watered them for a month or so, and then transplanted them. Over the coming years, I took great satisfaction in my little stand.

Fast-forward to 2014: on one memorable fall morning, I was charged with taking both our sons to school, which was a daylong commitment for me. I woke up with extreme anxiety. I was not even sure why. It was so extreme I wasn't sure how I would even get the boys to school, much less last all day there. I woke up early and had an extra forty-five minutes before our scheduled departure and knew I needed to do *something* to break that anxiety just a bit.

I took a short walk on our property, attempting to engage my brain in an adventure. I had spotted a quartz rock a couple of weeks prior, and I thought, "What if you find that rock again and turn it over to see if it has a vein of gold?" I headed out, exploring the wild west side of our property, found the rock, examined it carefully and didn't see the golden vein, and decided I would apparently find it in another rock. I was feeling a bit better, and so I considered the adventure a complete success. I walked back up to the house, right past the stand of lemon balm, and thought, "Wow, you're struggling with anxiety, and lemon balm is often recommended for anxiety!" I had never used lemon balm during an anxiety attack, but I reached down and picked a handful as I headed back to the house.

In the kitchen, as I packed the lunches for the day, I put the lemon balm in a large thermos and poured in boiling water. Throughout that cool fall day, I drank lemon balm tea from the thermos and enjoyed its soothing effect. I was struck by how powerful lemon balm is for anxiety. I was also struck by the realization that I had literally planted an anxiety remedy for myself some years before, on a good day.

What if on every single good day we establish structures for ourselves to make our inevitable bad days a little less bad? If we did this systematically and deliberately, how many more good days would accumulate as our bad days became less bad? It's a powerful idea and one that I would like to implement in my life even more deliberately and one that I can always improve on. (Someone should create an email course around that concept.)

Let's look at the same concept in the context of weight. We know that a major barrier each of us experiences to getting and staying trim relates to our mental health. Many of us are comfort eaters. Surely, we know this to be true on a basic level. When I hit maintenance, had some bad days, and struggled with eating comfort food, my struggle was easy to recognize. I was never a big binge eater nor an extreme comfort eater and so never appreciated the role mental health played in my struggle with food. I was a comfort eater pretty much like everyone else is: not so much of one that anyone ever recommended a therapist for it, but to be sure, I would overeat (and overdrink) when I was in a slump.

Here's the harsh truth: *It doesn't take much of a slump to stay fat or to get fat again.* That pint of premium ice cream is over 1,000 calories. A keto version may have a scant 800 calories. Each will put you up one-quarter to one-third of a pound of body fat. No one pint ever matters very much, which allows you to disassociate one pint at a time, not paying attention to its effect, right up to 300 pounds (136 kilograms) and higher up the scale, until you find yourself stuck, limping and lying around, unable to live your life as you want to.

What if we structured our eating strategically on good days to help us get through those inevitable bad days? What if we essentially set up Good Day Strategies to leverage on those bad days when we are at high risk of eating the pint of ice cream? How would our lives change? Would we, over months and then years of implementation, have fewer bad days?

Take a further step back. What if all the energy that we put into food went into something else, like hiking or crafting? How would a life full of hiking and crafting compare with a lifetime of struggle with obesity and comfort eating? What if your life was structured to favor hiking over eating that pint of ice cream? That is essentially the choice we have, a choice made clear by the many weight loss success cases in the Eat Like a Bear! community but a choice we each still struggle with individually. Structuring our lives so that we make the right choice is the key to long-term success. We struggle because while this Good Day Strategy idea and the RBS framework are both simple, they may also be the hardest things you're about to implement.

As you work on your implementation, lean into this meal framework, but not just because it meets the calorie-minded, carb-conscious, insulin-lowering conditions for weight loss but also because of its power as a Good Day Strategy. Therein we may find both the necessary and sufficient conditions for weight loss and weight maintenance.

BAD DAYS AND THE FOOD RULE

During my long grind of losing 140 pounds (64 kilograms), I developed another strategy for weigh loss called "make your food rule the night before." It took me at least two years of leading the Eat Like a Bear! community before I started paying attention to my personal psychology and how I structured my days. As I developed more psychology content for the community, I gradually became more aware of little behaviors of mine I had taken for granted.

Basically, every evening I make a concerted decision to eat a certain way the next day. Through all those months of dieting, my rule typically was "Eat one RBS each day and nothing more." (I didn't know then that it would be called the RBS, but you get what I mean.) I was flexible about this rule. If I had an upcoming event—such as a wedding or a potluck get-together—I would decide the night before how to handle the eating. I never allowed myself to decide in the moment, because that is, in fact, a scenario in which you are far more likely to eat the cookie or donut. I made my rule when I was strong, and I never broke my rule.

However, in maintenance I began to appreciate the boundary even more because I noticed that on bad days, especially if I allowed myself to eat in five hours, for instance, I struggled a good bit with not overeating. The harsh fact is that I could eat 5,000 calories in five hours. In fact, that would not even be difficult. On the bad days, I struggled and had to muster up additional restraint. As a result, not only were the bad days bad, but I was also, in effect, struggling more trying to live within that loosened boundary I had given myself.

Bad days became worse because of what I think of as "the long rope." I discuss this basic problem in a YouTube video and describe the maintenance problem of having too much rope. I compare the weight loss phase and maintenance to a dog on a leash. In weight loss, you've got a short little leash. Maintenance gives you a longer rope, but think about what happens to a dog on a longer rope: he gets wrapped around all the trees and bushes until he chokes himself on his collar.

The cold fact is this: *With too much rope in maintenance, some of us are going to find ourselves caught around that tree, gasping for air!* In fact, I've been on the razor's edge of undermining myself many times in maintenance, a point that I know so well that I have come to anticipate it and manage it.

For me, being stressed and busy with work or family is the greatest predictor of bad days, as it surely is with most of us. When I'm under stress, I'm likely to eat more. Also, stress raises cortisol, a hormone that encourages the body to store belly fat. With higher levels of fat hormones and a struggle with eating, I can easily gain 10 pounds or more over the course of a stressful month. I first became aware of the potential weight gain from stress during August and September 2020, which really challenged my mental and physical health. During that period, we implemented a lot of changes in our learning content and our email system at Eat Like a Bear!, all while appearing on the cover of *Woman's World* magazine.

After that challenging period of 2020, I looked back and applied my knowledge as I moved forward.

THE BAD DAYS AHEAD

As it would turn out, bigger challenges lay ahead in my life, and I survived by becoming more observant of myself and my own implementation of this way of eating. My first challenge would be in May 2021 when Eat Like a Bear! got super busy making plans to surprise our 100th Century Bear in Orlando. We keep a tally of people who have lost 100 pounds (45 kilograms) since finding us, and we affectionately call them Century Bears. As we were approaching the 100th Century Bear mark—the one hundredth person to lose 100 pounds in a year—we got the wild idea for the whole moderator team to surprise the Century Bear at home, in the style of Publishers Clearinghouse. (If you don't remember Publishers Clearinghouse, ask your mother or grandmother about it.)

What a great and completely crazy idea! We did it, and boy, I was busy and just pushed. My mother-in-law passed at the same time, and we were just stretched all over.

I had already recognized how I had struggled in August with the *Woman's World* publicity, especially the daily struggle with the eating boundary: it was always stressful to keep my eating in check. What I did in May 2021 instead was to go extra-strict. I committed to eating a calorie-restricted, one-meal RBS model every day for a month. I started that month with a puffy face from stress and spring allergies but ended the month slightly brighter, despite stress and high cortisol levels.

Interestingly, when I stepped back and surveyed that month, I realized my eating had been easier, not harder. I ate a good meal and walked away from food, focusing my brain on our Century Bear project. In fact, my whole month of stress was far easier simply because I did not have to fight with food—with all of the internal struggles to keep myself from eating more. I had a strict rule in place, and I followed it, just like the star student in school. Life as that star student during that busy month was far, far easier than it would have been.

May 2021 taught me this key point: if you can draw the line and walk away, life overall will be easier. If it then helps you reach your long-term goals and get out and live a vibrant life, then life is simply that much better overall. What I could not imagine in May 2021 is how much my learning that month would prepare me for six months hence.

At 6:51 p.m. on September 22, 2021, you would have found my son Alastair and me up on our house's highest roof watching in horror as a giant pyrocumulus cloud expanded over the eastern sky.

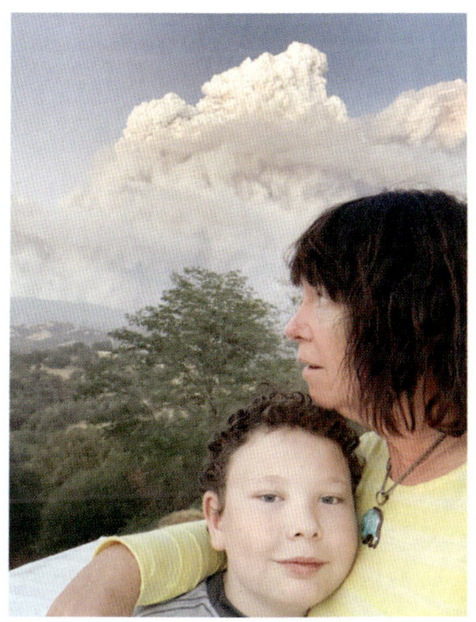

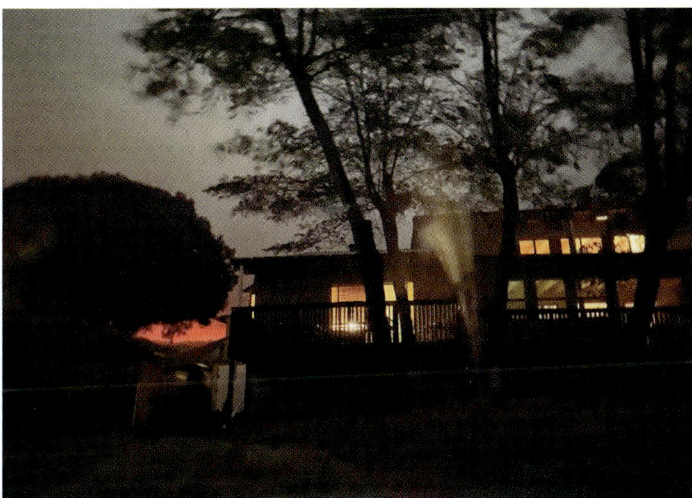

A pyrocumulus is a cloud caused by fire, usually an explosion of a huge amount of fuel, which often signals the beginning of the rapid expansion of a fire. The Windy Fire had been brewing north of us but jumped a line that September evening and barreled toward our house, taking groves of historic thousand-year-old giant sequoia trees with it.

The days of uncertainty during the evacuation were intense, but, so too, was the aftermath. If you've followed my weight loss story, you already know that a big part of my weight loss motivation was to get out and hike with my sons. In 2017, at my high weight of 280 pounds (127 kilograms), I was limping around my house with a knee injury, looking longingly at the giant sequoias from my window but unable to hike among them.

The forest here has been part of my own coping on bad days. On bad days, I would deliberately push myself out to hike, and I had certain rules: I would talk to people if I saw any, and I would look for a fragrant or edible plant to bring home for a project. I had built these coping structures over the years, but those structures and the world's most resilient trees were literally burned up in about two days' time. The giant sequoias that I could see on a distant ridge from my front deck in 2017 are now gone, as is much of the forest around them. My grief has been deep, and it has challenged my eating.

As I went through those difficult postfire months, I started to pay attention to the flow and emotions of my days. In that time, I noticed something extremely obvious that I've taken for granted all of these years; something I have never heard anyone talk about explicitly. It relates to the strategy "Eat and walk away." Let's look at two scenarios as an example.

On Roaming and Rummaging

Imagine two days where you end up eating the exact same thing, but on the first day you simply eat it and go on with your awesome scheduled activities. On the second day, you eat it and then fight with yourself all day long not to eat more. Your pants fit exactly the same after each of these days. Which day is better? We already know the answer. I had many days like these after the forest fire. I always made good eating decisions, but some days I struggled much more.

What happens when you do cave a little? To examine the consequences of caving, let's look at two parallel scenarios. Imagine waking up to a bad day, in each of two universes.

In universe one, you are completely prepared for the day. The day before you decided to make the Panang Chicken skillet dish, and you have all the ingredients ready. It may be a bad day, but you follow your plan when it is time to cook. You also have strategies ready for days like these: you know you always feel better if you spend time outdoors, so you push yourself out into your garden. It's not a great day, but it's surely not your worst day, either. You did it.

In universe two, you have no plan for the day. You have this very book on Ridiculously Big Skillets, and you know it works. You've stocked some ingredients for these dishes and have worked through the Six-Week Plan. But today, you are feeling so ho-hum that nothing sounds good.

You go to your freezer and ponder your options. Among some of the protein items you dutifully stashed in there, you also find two potpies and a frozen lasagna. Four days ago you had eyed these foods, but you had carefully avoided all of them. Today, as well, you grab the chicken strips instead, and you make Panang Chicken, but as you eat it, you think about those items in the freezer. As you eat the panang, you don't feel all that satisfied because you have already entertained the idea of lasagna and potpies. You rationalize to yourself that since you dutifully avoided these cheats four days ago, it's okay to eat just one small potpie today. After all, you are feeling so bad, surely it will help you feel just a little bit better.

That small potpie is a 600 calorie addition to your meal. If you added that every day to your eating, you would slow your weight loss by about six pounds a month (nearly three kilograms). You're aware that eating it adds calories, but you decide it's okay to eat it just this once since you don't eat it every day. You pop it in the microwave and eat it before thinking much more about it.

However, the bigger cost of the potpie is still to come. You eat it and then realize that you are still not satisfied and want another potpie. You can still taste the gravy, and so you struggle with yourself not to microwave a second. Then your whole internal battle begins where part of you wants a second potpie and part of you feels shame and guilt for the first potpie. There is no part of you actually happy or satisfied as you sit and ponder the second potpie. The you in universe one has cut thoughts of food and is now gardening, while in universe two you are upset about potpies.

You struggle, but you remember the directive in this book: "Eat and walk away." You finally push yourself to your garden. You have escaped your freezer roaming with "only" 600 extra calories. It could have been far worse. But what was the psychological cost to you that you paid for those 600 calories? How much effort was it for you to avoid eating an additional 1,200 calories?

Imagine an entire year in universe one. Imagine an entire year in universe two. Which universe would you choose to live in? What is actually required to live in the much more straightforward universe one with a straighter path to your long-term goal?

BECOME A MEAL-CRAFTING TECHNOCRAT

In my months in the aftermath of the forest fire, I played right in the middle of those two universes, doing pretty well at not eating the proverbial potpie. But I noticed something pretty powerful: not having a very clear intention and boundary on what I would eat made my day that much harder.

As I look back on my own long grind in 2017–2018 and the 140 pounds I lost, I am struck by the mental game I played with myself: I approached the food each day like a technocrat, like a person tasked with food managerial efficiency. My purpose was to craft a tasty meal but one within the boundaries that would help me reach my long-term goals. My meals had no other purpose.

Because of my overall mindset, I woke up every day in universe one. Yes, some days were good, and on those good days I might experiment a bit more with adding fresh herbs to my dish or roasting vegetables. On bad days, I woke up with the same technocratic approach, and this approach forestalled any roaming of the freezer or refrigerator or visit to a drive-through fast-food joint and any subsequent struggle I might have over straying from my path. Meal-crafting technocrats win the long game because they don't roam on those bad days.

Examining my case through this lens, I would argue that a key factor in my own success in 2017 is that I put my technocratic self in charge. I worked to prove to myself that I had done everything I could do to lose weight, and I charged my scientific self with that task. Scientists gather feedback and make changes based on objective data. Scientists often make excellent technocrats and are prepared to replicate their experiments with precision every single day.

Putting my inner technocrat completely in charge of my eating may have been the best Good Day Strategy I ever subconsciously implemented. My bad days were just that much easier when the technocratic part of me was in charge of the food.

RBS SUCCESS IS 90 PERCENT A HEAD GAME

For at least a year and a half I have wondered how much the effectiveness of the RBS method lies in the specifics of the ingredients and how much lies in the psychology. With the struggles I faced in 2021 myself,

I'm inclined to put the psychology part at more than 90 percent of the effectiveness.

All the internal struggle that you feel—that internal negotiation that I discuss in some of my psychology content—we all go through it. It is something that is described in detail in the social choice theory I learned in my political science graduate school days, a theoretical framework I applied to voting and public opinion in the 1990s. Meanwhile, a small group of theorists was applying social choice theory to weight loss and addiction—while we focused instead on voting, while getting fatter and straining our livers.

Do you know that feeling when you've struggled your whole life with your weight and fear getting fat again? That struggle you feel, especially on your bad days as you make bad decisions and then start down that whole road of self-doubt and second-guessing, takes a whole lot of energy. Internal turmoil is turmoil that you cannot escape.

That turmoil can be caused by something as simple as a handful of almonds, and almonds are even healthy. There is nothing really wrong with almonds. The problem is that, without boundaries, a little snack of eight almonds can quickly become two cups of almonds when we don't pay attention. So there we are on that long rope trying to eat just eight almonds, and the turmoil begins: Should I have eaten those extra nuts? Will that handful of nuts today become three handfuls tomorrow? How soon will I need to shop for larger pants? Those almonds plague us nearly every waking moment. They may plague us in our sleep, as well. They're an example, a giant symbol, of how we ended up fat in the first place.

If this all sounds dramatic and extreme to you, then I direct you to the jar of almonds. For most of the rest of us, I direct you to the boundaries you can embrace in the RBS framework. The ingredients of the RBS may be necessary for weight loss, but they are not likely sufficient. The approach we take in implementation hopefully provides us with sufficient conditions.

For those of you who have waited months for this book, you can see why I have hesitated to publish a "collection of recipes." Anyone who views this book as just a recipe collection probably has the necessary but not sufficient conditions for weight loss. The world surely has enough weight loss books that don't actually work.

The success you see in the community with the RBS model comes from the ingredient list *and* from how it is implemented. Survey our success cases. Shine a bright light into their minds, and you will likely see a lot of psychology baked into their implementation in ways they are likely not even cognizant of. Some of them are struggling in maintenance as they work to unwrap that proverbial long rope from the bushes.

Here's your core task: implement these skillet recipes, but if you are seeking a recipe to save you from your struggle with weight, let's do it right. Let's not view this as some sort of magical solution. The RBS framework, raw or cooked, works not just because of its calorie-minded, low-carb, filling nature but also because of the structural boundaries you set to turn up the heat on your own head game. On your good days, engage deeply in the RBS framework so that you are ready on those bad days to implement it like a pro.

chapter two

The RBS Framework: When and What to Eat

WHEN TO EAT

I am a time-restricted eater, which means that I eat all of my nutrition for the day in a small window of time. In my rapid weight loss phase, I ate one Ridiculously Big Salad in one hour. In maintenance, I have played around with some loosened versions of the same framework: two smaller meals in five hours, for instance. Both are examples of time-restricted eating. Eating in the narrower window of time is a more intensive approach to weight loss.

I have long attributed the "when to eat" aspect of all of this as the game-changer for me, and for the most part, it was, but my reasons have come to evolve.

When I first started the community, I was focused on the food and nutrition part of what we do, assuming that my specific nutritional choices were the key to my success. The main new eating structure I had implemented was the time-restricted eating portion, and so I have attributed much of my success to the biological reasoning behind time-restricted eating. If we limit the hours in which we eat, we limit our body's production of insulin. Excessive insulin makes us fat, and if our body is producing insulin all day long because we snack all day long, we might just find our weight continuing to creep up.

Restricting our eating to a smaller window of hours each day most definitely has a positive biological effect on weight loss. Do not overlook that key point. However, it is also easy to focus on the nutritional aspect of what we are doing and miss some critical elements.

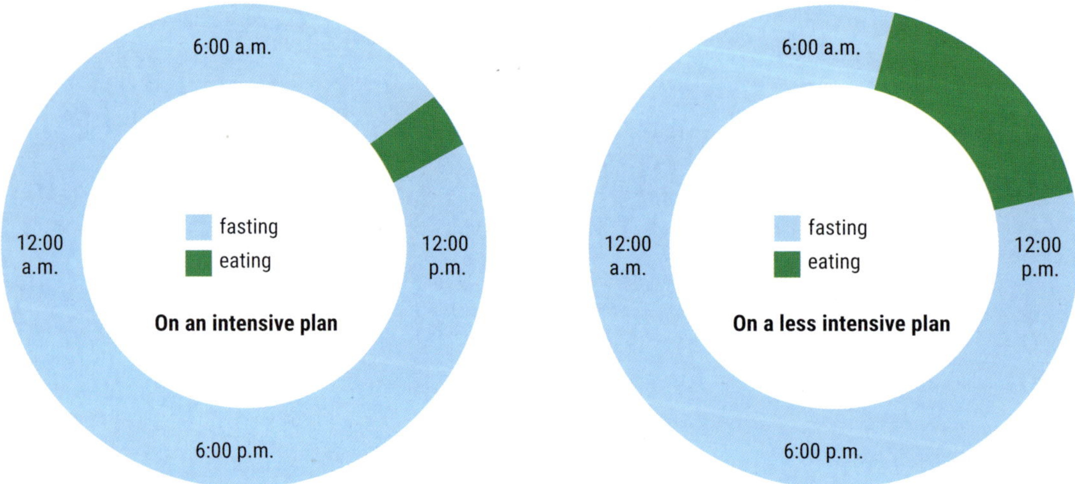

Here's what I have learned over five years of weight loss and maintenance: with more mindful mental discipline, eating within a narrow window of the day both reduces my production of insulin *and* allows me to walk away from food for twenty or more hours at a time. When I walk away from food, a crazy thing happens: I think less about food, I eat less, and I think far less about the food I should not have eaten because, in fact, I didn't eat the food.

Aggregate all of that "food thinking" and "food worrying" over many hours and many days and that time-restricted eating framework just changed your life, only in small part because of its effect on your insulin production.

I realize that eating in just a few hours a day may sound radical and perhaps overly austere. I definitely have people respond to my austerity with great sympathy: they feel sorry for me, living with what appears to be deep asceticism. However, personally I have never been so satisfied with life as I am today. I had not appreciated the energy it drained from me all of those years worrying about whether my pants still fit (and, in fact, they often did not).

WHAT TO EAT

When I first started the Eat Like a Bear! community, I gave people the food list that is at the end of this chapter and told people to shoot for the green zone. The foods in that zone are lower in carbohydrates and less likely to spike your insulin than foods with more sugars. It was good advice, and people had success with it, but the community's success improved as my recommendations got more specific. My own meals fit with my recommendations but were actually much more specific, which community members started noticing. One member, Nancy, called me out and wanted to know *exactly* what I was eating. As I mentioned previously, I was struck by the framework nature of my eating once I took to replicating and measuring my meals one year later.

As I write in *Half My Size with the Ridiculously Big Salad,* the RBS has three core parts and an optional fourth part for added flavor and texture. In the remainder of this chapter, I give you an overview of how to put these parts together.

RBS Part 1: Lots and Lots of Vegetables

If the basis of the classic RBS is the greens, that of our cooked dishes is the cooked vegetables. The vegetable could be a cooked green, such as cabbage or kale, but it could also be cauliflower, broccoli, okra, green beans, or any of the lower-carb vegetables.

Some people try right away to fine-tune the classic RBS by refining the base, such as choosing to eat only greens that are organic, wild harvested, or locally sourced from the farmers' market, and you may be inclined to do the same with the cooked vegetables in these cooked recipes. But I encourage you to keep it simple and not get too hung up on the type and source of your vegetables. First, learn the framework and make the meal as simple as possible so that you can easily and quickly implement it on your inevitable bad days. On your bad days, you are not likely to shop at the farmers' market and then carefully process your organic vegetables into one of these meals. On those bad days, you have to resist the temptation of the fast-food drive-through.

Key to the framework is keeping plenty of frozen vegetables on hand. I am not suggesting that you only eat frozen never fresh, but it's an easy go-to source for those bad days or days when you are in a rush. It's also important to eat a variety of vegetables, which is easier to do if you fill your freezer with a wide selection. Over time, you will learn what you like so you can stock your freezer with those favored vegetables.

The recipes in this book rely on the most commonly available frozen vegetables. They do not include root vegetables, such as potatoes, which are high in carbohydrates, nor difficult-to-source frozen items, like artichoke hearts. If you have access to these more unusual items and they fit your groove, you can surely craft recipes around them. Feel free to modify the vegetable base portion of these recipes to your liking, being mindful to avoid or minimize high-carb vegetables.

The recipes use 12 ounces (340 grams) of vegetables, because frozen vegetables commonly come in 12-ounce packages. However, in practice, my own cooked meals range from 8 to 16 ounces (225 to 450 grams), depending on my hunger and the size of the freezer bag. I often buy 32-ounce bags of broccoli, for instance, and typically use half in a dish. I could use one-third instead—but you will never find me measuring 12 ounces (340 grams) out of that 32-ounce bag (900 grams). Don't get hung up on the exact amount: eat whatever amount you need to fill you up and get you to tomorrow.

RBS Part 2: The Fat and Flavor of the Sauce

All the sauces in this book are in the range of 400 to 500 calories. The main ingredients for some of the sauces are lower in calories, and for those, I've added cheese or sour cream, which are added at the end so they do not curdle. If you want to trim down these recipes to a lower-calorie version, simply eliminate the dairy wherever it appears.

Most of these recipes include 50 grams or more of fat. That's a pretty good bit of fat in a meal that is otherwise highly calorie minded, but the fat will help you stay satiated. At the same time, these meals are low enough in fat that your body will shift to living off your stored fat. (Some years ago in a live video, someone asked about the difficulty of sitting with her family during a meal and not eating. I responded: "You're sitting on your food!" That quote stuck.)

Keep in mind that the sauce is there to make the meal flavorful and satisfying enough that you can take pleasure in it—and then draw the line and walk away from food for the day.

RBS Part 3: The Protein on Top

You may have guessed from some of my recipes and videos that I am not a measurer or macro counter. When people ask: "How much protein do you eat?" I stumble around searching for an answer because my mind just wants to blurt out: "I eat whatever I feel like." My protein intake does vary, and I make no effort to measure it or to eat in a certain framework of macro intake, which is common in the world of ketogenic diets. However, all my meals do include a significant amount of protein. Nutritionists commonly recommend eating a portion of protein about the size of a deck of cards twice daily, which roughly equates to 6 ounces of meat (180 grams of meat by weight). I typically eat about two decks or 6 to 8 ounces a day (180 to 225 grams of meat by weight). Note that this is a ballpark measure of the weight of the meat, not the grams of actual

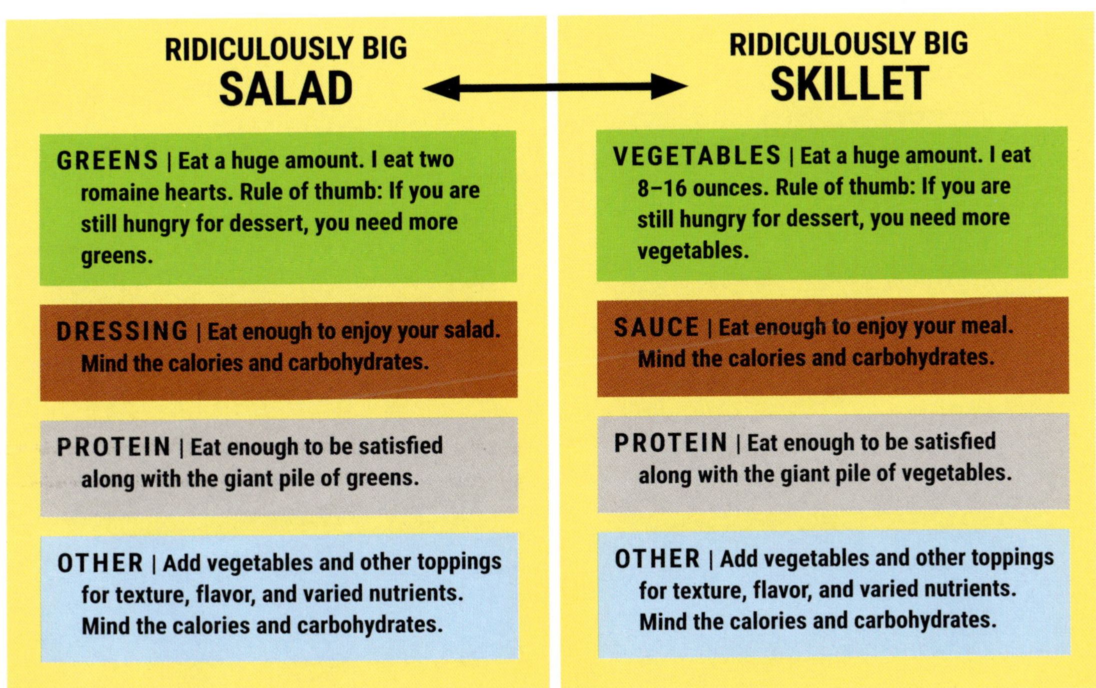

protein in the meat. For example, 100 grams of beef by weight has about 25 grams of protein. I do not actually count either one but include the weight of the protein part of these dishes to help get you in range.

As you eat your meals, you will probably figure out about how much protein you need to feel satisfied. In the keto world, some experts get concerned that people on these diets are eating too much protein. I am not sure where the research will land on this one, and I do not really

RBS FRAMEWORK FAQS

Is it healthy to eat processed meat?
As with all food, your best long game play is to eat whole foods. However, this book does include sausage and bacon for added flavor and convenience. Do not center all of your eating on these items, and select specific products that have little or no added sugars.

Should I weigh my protein before or after it is cooked?
For the most part, I eat the equivalent of a couple of decks of cards (about 180 grams), and I eyeball that amount when the protein is cooked. There is little difference in the leaner meats. For fatty meat such as ground beef, I tend to drain the fat and focus on the meat. In that case, I am counting the cooked and drained meat on my plate.

What if I eat too much protein?
In the context of these meals, I would not be concerned about adding additional unprocessed protein if you are craving it. With the dishes in this book and the original RBS book, the protein is balanced well with the vegetable component. As with all ingredients, do consider the calories of what you are adding in light of your goals. If you find yourself in a protein-craving phase, you might consider some of the leaner meats like shrimp or skinless chicken breasts.

What if I don't like broccoli (or cauliflower or green beans)?
As you learn the framework, simply mix and match ingredients to suit your tastes.

What if I eat a plant-based diet?
Replace the meat and dairy options with plant-based alternatives, being mindful of the carbohydrate content and added sugar. Your meals will be higher in carbs but probably far better for weight loss than what you are currently eating. If you cut the dairy items in these meals, you might need to replace them with higher-calorie and high-fat foods like nuts and avocados to make a more satisfying and filling meal.

What if I am not quite full with this meal?
I do find the RBS skillet meals to be a bit less filling than the raw salads, and as a result, I tend to include strategies to help bring me to fullness faster. One trick is to swig a couple of ounces of apple cider vinegar (diluted in a few ounces of water) as you prepare your meal. For some people, this reduces their appetite. In addition, you can thicken your meals with glucomannan powder, which also helps with fullness. Drink seltzer with your meal. The bubbles in the seltzer will expand in your stomach and likely make you feel fuller, too.

Finally, add some cabbage to the dish. Cabbage may be the most filling vegetable, raw or cooked. It is also mild in flavor and can be added easily to any of these dishes while adding negligible calories.

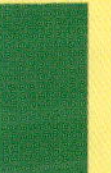

EAT BEARISHLY: leafy greens; unprocessed meat, fish, and seafood; eggs; non-root vegetables; coffee; tea; stevia and monk fruit (sweeteners); oils (olive, coconut, avocado).

EAT WITH RESTRAINT: processed meat (read labels); dairy (cheese, yogurt, sour cream, etc.: read labels); nuts and seeds, berries, and condiments (read labels or make your own); root vegetables, beans and legumes, whole grains (read labels).

DO NOT EAT: sugared drinks, juice, coffee "creamer," alcohol, white flour products (e.g., bread, pasta, crackers, pretzels), potatoes and related products (e.g., chips, fries), breakfast cereal.

WHEN TO EAT: reduce your eating window. Give your body's hormones a rest. I eat in 1 hour each day. Keep your eating in 8 hours or less. Eat in 5 hours (or 1 hour!) for better results.

SNACKS: CUT THEM OUT. If you're eating in a larger window (5–8 hours), try eating two distinct meals and cutting out the snacks in between. Even a snack will affect your insulin level.

worry about it, because the huge amount of vegetables you have along with your protein really does limit your protein intake. If you eat all the vegetables, you simply will not have room in your stomach for a huge amount of protein. That said, on days when I seem to be craving protein, I eat more. I cannot imagine that a protein craving is a bad craving, and so I go with it.

RBS Part 4: The Other Stuff

Your basic cooked RBS has vegetables, a sauce, and a protein. To round out the flavor and texture of your meal, you may choose to add other items, such as nuts or cream. I think it's great to add to the dishes in this book, but just be aware of what you are adding and make sure those additions will help you meet your bigger goals.

Whenever you add an item, you add more calories, so be mindful, particularly if you have a lot of weight to lose. You could easily add one-quarter cup of cream to any of these dishes, which seems like a small amount. However, that quarter cup is an additional 200 calories, which could reduce your weight loss by about 2 pounds a month (nearly a kilogram). Certainly, many people can consume more calories in a day than this strict model I am suggesting and still manage to lose weight. If that is you and you want to splurge a bit, go for it.

If you are new to learning about the carbohydrates and calories in foods, a food app might be in order to help you get started. The three-zone food list may help as well. Depending on your weight loss goals, you may only need to cut out the biggest offenders in red, or you may need to be more intensive and stick pretty strictly to the green zone.

SUPPLEMENTS AND ELECTROLYTES

All readers of this book who see a doctor for kidney or cardiac issues, or perhaps anything requiring a specialist, will want to check in with their doctor about electrolytes. If you are restricted in your sodium due to hypertension, for instance, do follow your doctor's advice, and pay no attention to the rest of this sidebar article. Anyone on dialysis should not even consider reading the rest of this sidebar.

For those of us in good health, there is no supplement that is required for success, given the nutrient density and variety of the meals we tend to eat. Some people do take a daily multi-vitamin, mindful of the possible added sugar. However, we may find ourselves at times needing some added electrolyte minerals, especially while transitioning into this way of eating or while engaged in more rigorous physical activities.

If you are just getting started with this way of eating, take note of what is commonly called "the keto flu" and the relief you may get from added electrolytes. The keto flu is simply a set of flu-like symptoms that come as your body adapts to a new lower-carbohydrate diet. If you have been eating a diet high in carbohydrates, you are more likely to be affected by the fluish symptoms of dizziness, nausea, and leg cramps as you transition away from the carbohydrates.

These fluish symptoms are most likely to hit as you are getting started, for a number of reasons, but this is the most compelling: We all tend to lose a bit of water weight at the beginning of our weight loss phase. Those fluids we lose contain minerals, and when those fluids get flushed out of our bodies, so do the minerals. All that water weight was a mineral storage for us, and that mineral storage is suddenly gone. What a shock that can be to our bodies! The headache and nausea set in as we adjust.

Over the long term, we can get these minerals from a healthy diet, rich in vegetables, but often dietary minerals are not quite enough in the early phase of a low-carbohydrate way of eating. In addition, as the weeks and months pass and you become more active and engage in more rigorous outdoor activities, especially in the heat, you may need more electrolytes.

As you shop for electrolytes, you will see products vary a lot in the amount of sodium, potassium, magnesium, and other minerals they supply. Ratios of those minerals also vary a lot. Homemade recipes in our own Eat Like a Bear! community vary a lot.

Do you know what else varies a lot?

Each of our individual needs for sodium, potassium, and magnesium.

Our needs vary because of our own slightly different physiologies but also because we each have varying amounts of these minerals in our diets.

What do we do?

As for an app, any popular app will do, but some risk overly complicating your eating. For instance, Carb Manager, which emphasizes a very low carb, keto diet, is popular and can be useful in some cases. However, according to Carb Manager, all the meals in this book are over the carb limit—and so your risk is that the robot on your mobile phone may cause you to doubt your own common sense. Carb Manager has not actually ever lost any weight itself, so do keep in mind the wisdom of following robots. A basic calorie-counting app like Simple Calorie Counter may be a better choice.

As you get started, you may have a headache, nausea, or dizziness that might respond quite readily to added sodium, potassium, and magnesium. Be ready with a supplement.

You can buy or make your own electrolyte mix and use this conservative strategy of dosing: If, after a basic daily dose, your symptoms are alleviated, then you are consuming enough. If the supplemental minerals helped but you still have some symptoms, consider adding an additional drink for a few days. If your symptoms do not respond to the electrolytes, check in with your doctor. You could have the actual flu or some other malady.

BUY THEM

For a premade electrolyte powder, seek out suggestions in the Eat Like a Bear! community. I hesitate to make a brand recommendation in print since formulations do change. We have had many requests over the years for us to provide an electrolyte product. Perhaps we will even be organized enough one day to craft a cool one for you.

MAKE YOUR OWN

In my own house, I keep powder forms of sodium ascorbate, potassium chloride, and magnesium citrate to mix up a portion when I am more active, particularly in the summer.

These days, I do not take these supplemental minerals daily, but I do take them when I am under unusual stress, especially from the heat.

I also notice that in the summertime I tend to add a lot of salt to my meals. I am inclined to follow my instincts on the sodium and add as much salt to my meal as I want. We have many recipes in the group that are much higher in sodium, but those levels simply may not be necessary if we are all keeping a salt shaker handy at mealtime and just lean into our taste buds. (Again, people under medical directive to reduce their salt intake should not have read that last sentence.)

That said, I do whip up a drink in my kitchen to have for those hot summer days. It is also a very good starting place if you are at risk of "keto flu."

I make a little powder mixture with ratios that are approximately these: 100–200 mg sodium ascorbate, 200–500 mg potassium chloride, and 100–200 mg magnesium citrate.

I add my powder concoction to about 2 cups of water. Some days, I admit that I do drink my electrolytes in one sitting. Some people end up with gastric distress if they do so, so you may want to sip your beverage over some hours, just in case.

chapter three

The Super Simple Approach for Your Ridiculously Big Skillet

If you have not noticed already, I will again highlight the point that every recipe in this book relies on either frozen vegetables or washed and bagged greens. Each uses powdered seasonings. This is by design, and it actually took a good bit of effort to make these recipes this simple.

Developing a cookbook with recipes for these soups, skillets, and sautés began in the days before the COVID-19 quarantine. I was joined by Anna Sul and her children, all of whom are talented cooks. We set up shop at at a school near the foothills of the Sierra Nevada mountains in central California, gathering for the first time on a Friday in March 2020 to test recipes. We made dishes in the kitchen of the school's parent lounge and served them up to the administrators and any other drop-ins who showed up on the school grounds that day, when no classes were in session. We held mini taste tests with these embarrassingly simple recipes until we felt that we had a handle on what we call the "skillet recipes" in this book.

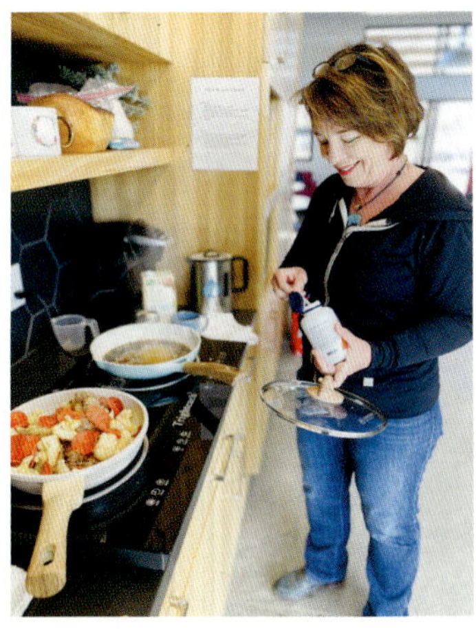

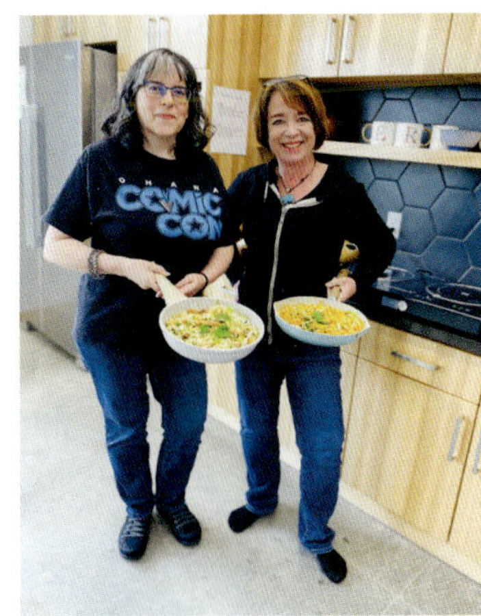

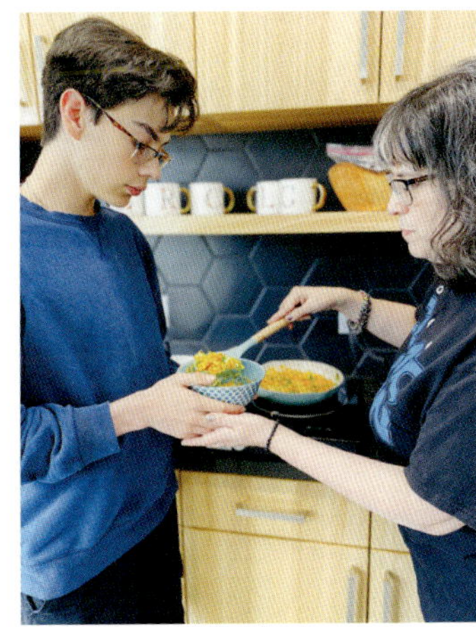

It's a good thing that we are pretty scrappy and adept cooks, because the school was about to close for more than a year due to COVID, and we lost our ready-made taste-test community. Even with a swift start, it would take us eighteen months to create recipes that we might otherwise have created in three months had we not lost our access to the school's kitchen and staff.

All of us on the school grounds that day knew how to cook, and we each had to get over ourselves to get these recipes right. My big barrier was basically getting over my own preconception that if you were writing a book with recipes, those recipes ought to be gourmet and use the best-quality ingredients.

The hallmark of the RBS, cooked or not, and the success of the original book, *Half My Size with the Ridiculously Big Salad,* is due in large part to the extreme simplicity of the recipes. We realized that when you start preparing a cooked meal, it is easy to get complicated quickly, and so we challenged ourselves at each step to make the recipes as easy as possible. We knew they needed to be simpler than anything you would ever find in any cookbook out there, and they needed to compete timewise with the frozen fast food in your freezer.

As we tested recipes, our conversations went something like this:

"Maybe we don't need to sauté the garlic and seasonings in oil. Why not just dump them all in?" "That's good, but what if we replace the fresh garlic with powdered garlic?"

That was a breakthrough moment for those of us who were used to fresh garlic, which happened to be all of us that day.

You are free, of course, to level-up any of the recipes that you find in here. I leave you to that task of roasting the vegetables or sautéing fresh garlic and ginger. But do not overlook the benefit of simplicity or view it as a deficit. Embrace the approach, because there will be days you will need it, even if you tend to be the person who always uses fresh garlic.

BE PREPARED

If you have all your ingredients at hand, your soup, skillet, or sauté will take less than 10 minutes to prepare and about 20 minutes to cook. That's it.

Your core points of preparation are these:

- Have basic seasonings available in your pantry.
- Keep a supply of frozen vegetables handy.
- Keep broth available in some fashion, either cartons of broth that you purchase or frozen homemade broth.
- Have a supply of protein items available, either in your freezer that you cook or purchased precooked.
- Keep a few other ingredients handy, such as cheese or sour cream, if you tend to use them in these dishes.

Remember that it's important to always be ready in case you wake up to an extra-bad day. Be prepared so that you can take care of the eating business without relying on takeout or other conveniences.

BEGIN YOUR PROTEIN PREPARATION

Your protein organization and preparation is the linchpin to implementing all of this in an easy and highly replicable fashion. There are all sorts of ways to go about it, but I highly encourage you to grab one little idea here and start it right now.

This is such a simple part of this book, and there is no way that this idea is unique, but the approach I have come to use for protein preparation and storage is seen by many readers of *Half My Size with the Ridiculously Big Salad* as a game-changing strategy in their own kitchen preparation. Do give this section some thought. The method may be game-changing for you as well, or perhaps spur you into an even better idea.

First, as you will see, you can buy a whole lot of these protein items conveniently cooked for you. They cost a bit more, and you need to do some checking to make sure they have not added a bunch of sugar or some other ingredient you are avoiding. However, there is no reason these days that you need to cook your own chicken strips if you've got the money to pay a big chicken place to do it for you. That is certainly an option. I use a mixed strategy, depending mostly on the ebb and flow of my life. Do what works for you.

The basic idea for preparing protein is very simple: I cook a giant batch of protein, season it lightly, and then divide it into meal-size portions and freeze them. If you normally cook for two, freeze sizes accordingly. Label the bag with the contents and date. The key concept is that you are batch-cooking protein, lightly seasoned and ready to use, and then freezing it in portion sizes that are most useful to you.

Seasoning your meat lightly at this stage gives you the flexibility of using it in many different recipes. However, if you always use the meat for a specific purpose, then consider seasoning it accordingly. For example, I keep cooked ground beef with taco seasoning to use in Mexican-inspired dishes. I also keep ground beef seasoned with only salt and pepper. If I run out of taco meat, I can use the lightly seasoned ground beef in Mexican dishes simply by adding some taco seasoning.

Experiment with your most useful storage size. I typically fill freezer bags with the amount of protein I tend to use in one ridiculously big serving. When it is time for me to eat, I simply remove it from the freezer, rip open the bag, and place the frozen item on top of my warming skillet for hot skillet dishes. For salads, I use the same basic strategy but just defrost the protein alone in the skillet as I put the salad together.

Tip: Flatten out the freezer baggies before you freeze them. Do not load them so much that you can't flatten them. You want to be able to stack these baggies like a tower in your freezer.

What follows are quick tips for buying and processing meat and seafood. There are an endless number of cuts as well as devices to cook them. As you find cuts available to you, just do an internet search for the basic approach to cooking that item as you intend to cook it: "How to roast chicken in an Instant Pot." "How to smoke pork in a smoker." "How to make roast beef in an oven."

In fact, what you can do right after you read this is hit the store and buy a meat cut or buy some of this stuff cooked for you and then just cherry-pick through some recipes in this book to get started.

Chicken and Turkey Preparation

You can walk into nearly any store these days and purchase cooked chicken strips or a rotisserie chicken. That is always an option. You can even make broth from the bones of a rotisserie chicken using the instructions in this chapter. You can also certainly do what our mothers did and cook chicken or turkey yourself.

As convenient as chicken strips are in particular, they are also relatively expensive and hurt my frugal heart. You can watch for sales of raw chicken strips and then simply cook them yourself. If you go this direction, I tend to buy 3 to 4 pounds at a time, cook it all up, and serve a portion of it to my family that day. I freeze the rest in serving-size freezer baggies.

Roasting in the oven may still be the most common way to cook something like chicken breasts, but if you have a pressure cooker, grill, or smoker, those are great options as well, with instructions just an internet search away.

Don't overlook turkey, especially in postholiday sales. You can use turkey in any of the chicken recipes in this book.

Chicken Breasts in the Oven

1. **Preheat.** Preheat the oven to 425°F (220°C). Place a baking rack in the middle of the oven.
2. **Oil and season.** Rub avocado oil on the chicken breasts. Sprinkle on a basic all-purpose seasoning, giving them a good dusting (about ¼ teaspoon [1 ml] per breast if you are measuring, a light dusting if you are not). Place the breasts on a baking sheet lined with parchment paper or silicone.
3. **Roast.** Roast the chicken, uncovered, for 30 to 40 minutes. Check for doneness beginning at 30 minutes, using a meat

thermometer to check for an internal temperature of 165°F (74°C). A thorough food safety person would check the thickest part of the breast and would test each breast, ensuring they are all completely, safely cooked.

4. **Cool.** When done, allow the chicken to cool before freezing.
5. **Cut or shred as desired.** Before you freeze the breasts, you might cut them to size according to your intended use, though whole breasts freeze very well.
6. **Freeze.** Place in freezer baggies in amounts appropriate for your meals. Flatten, label, and stack in the freezer.

Beef Preparation

As with chicken, precooked beef strips are becoming commonplace in supermarkets, also with a premium markup but most definitely convenient for our purposes. Buy some of those if you are pressed for time and just getting started.

If leaning into those precooked steak strips hurts your frugal heart, as it does mine, most definitely shop for sales on beef cuts and batch-cook the heck out of them. As with the chicken, a quick internet search for the cut and your cooking device is your best method for implementation (e.g., "How to grill tri tip." "How to cook chuck roast in a slow cooker"). The combinations of cuts and cooking devices are fairly endless. The internet solution really shines in this instance.

Ground beef is as common in my kitchen, nearly as common as hydrogen is in the universe. I buy at least five pounds at a time and form part of it into burger patties, which I feed to my crew. The rest I cook up using the following basic cooking process, yielding some lightly seasoned ground beef. Sometimes I will use taco seasoning if I want to freeze meat with the flavor of Mexican cuisine. Any path will do: you can freeze it lightly seasoned and then add more flair to it when you complete your recipe. Do what works in your own kitchen.

Ground Beef on the Stove Top

1. **Heat the skillet.** Start heating the skillet on high.
2. **Add oil for lean meats.** If you are using a leaner meat, add a table-

spoon (15 ml) or two of a high-heat oil (e.g., avocado oil) to the skillet.

3. **Cook.** Add ground meat to the hot skillet, using a spatula to break it up a bit. Continue to break it up as it cooks, about every 2 minutes. Cook for about 8 minutes.
4. **Season.** Add about ½ tablespoon (7 ml) of an all-purpose seasoning per pound (450 g) of meat. Stir well. Adjust for salt and pepper.
5. **Consider draining the fat.** You can end up with a whole lot of fat in these skillets with ground beef. If you keep it, consider it as some of the fat in the sauce. You may not need to add fat to the sauce in your dish.
6. **Cool.** Allow the meat to cool before storing in the freezer.
7. **Freeze.** Place in freezer baggies in amounts appropriate for your meals. Flatten, label, and stack in the freezer.

Pork Preparation

The world of pork offers a whole lot of options in the "cooked for you" category. Sausage and ham are both ready-made convenience foods. You can buy a giant ham on sale after the holidays and divide it into freezer bags for longer-term storage. Of course, there is also sausage that you need to cook yourself, in which case you can cook it up on your stove top pretty readily and batch-freeze whatever you do not eat that day.

There are cooked pork products out there, like pulled pork, that are only lightly seasoned (and not smothered in a sugary barbecue sauce). There are also low-carbohydrate sauces available commercially. Hunt around for convenient pork products if you use pork on your dishes.

Pork Roast in the Pressure Cooker

1. **Season the meat.** Sprinkle on an all-purpose seasoning on the roast, giving it a good dusting (about 1 tablespoon per pound [30 ml per kg] if you are measuring, a light dusting if you are not). Place the roast on a trivet (particularly if the roast is frozen) in the pressure cooker.

2. **Moisten.** Add 2 cups (470 ml) of broth or water to the pressure cooker. You can use any sort of bone broth you have, even if the bone type does not match the meat type you are cooking. It will simply add more flavor. Water works, too; it just does not have the additional flavor.
3. **Seal.** Close and seal the pressure cooker. Check the vent to make sure it is set to "seal."
4. **Cook.** Set on manual using these guidelines: 70 minutes for 2 pounds (1 kg) and 80 minutes for 3 pounds (1.4 kg). Add 10 minutes per additional pound (½ kg).
5. **Release.** When the timer beeps and the meat has been cooked, use the manual release option to release the steam and slow the additional cooking process.
6. **Cool.** Remove the meat from the pot to cool it more quickly. Slice or shred the roast.
7. **Freeze.** Place in freezer baggies in amounts appropriate for your meals. Flatten, label, and stack in the freezer.

Seafood and Fish Preparation

There are a lot of options out there for cooked fish and seafood. Cooking instructions are highly variable across seafood types, which is partly why many recipes do not include them. Preparation methods vary depending on whether you are adding cooked shrimp to a skillet dish or using frozen raw fish, such as frozen salmon fillets. You can, in fact, find many simple options to add to these dishes, but you might find them best cooked separately and added to your dish later. Both scallops and shrimps can end up overcooked if they are cooked along with the other ingredients in the dish. It is better to cook them on the side and add them at the end.

If you are purchasing raw seafood or fish to batch-cook and freeze, your most likely choice is a fillet of some kind. Grilled or smoked fish are delicious, but most of us are more likely to pop fish in the oven or cook it in a skillet.

Salmon Fillets in the Oven

1. **Preheat.** Preheat your oven to 450°F (230°C).
2. **Season.** Season the salmon with an all-purpose seasoning, about a teaspoon per pound (5 ml per ½ kg) or a dusting across the fillets.
3. **Skin down.** Place on a baking sheet, skin side down if your salmon has skin.
4. **Bake.** Bake for 12 to 15 minutes, until the salmon is cooked through. It will flake with a fork when it is done. (When white goo comes out of the side of the fillets, it is overcooked but most definitely still edible. The white stuff is just albumin and a signal to turn your oven down just a touch next time and perhaps check the salmon a minute or two earlier.)
5. **Cool.** Allow the salmon to cool before freezing.
6. **Freeze.** Place in freezer baggies in amounts appropriate for your meals. Flatten, label, and stack in the freezer.

Protein Preparation for Vegetarians and Vegans

As a nod to our Veggie Bear community, I'm including a protein preparation section for vegetarians.

It has been twenty-five years since my vegetarian days, and I am amazed at all of the options out there these days. There are various meat replacements that mimic beef, pork, chicken, and turkey, and they are flavored with the sorts of seasonings we associate with steak and sausage. You can obviously use these items to replace the meats I use in my dishes. As with any processed food, compare ingredients and, in particular, find those with little or no added sugar. Look for foods that have fewer unpronounceable ingredients (an important point with any food we buy). These products often come frozen in meal-size portions.

Other common protein sources for vegetarians are fermented soybean products, such as tofu and tempeh, and seitan, or "wheat meat," a wheat protein. Though tempeh is traditionally fermented from soybeans, a variety of soy-free tempehs are available, made from chickpeas, lentils, and beans (black, mung, kidney, etc.). Note that one block or package of tofu has about 32 grams of protein.

All these products freeze well; in fact, some people prefer cooking with tofu that has been frozen. The tofu attains a spongy texture and absorbs sauces more readily. To freeze tofu, slice a block of extra-firm tofu into ½-inch slices, spread them on a plate or baking sheet, and freeze overnight. Put the frozen slices in freezer baggies in meal-size portions and store in the freezer. The frozen tofu keeps for up to a month.

Vegetarians, unlike vegans, have the obvious protein choices of eggs and dairy items, along with plant proteins. (For more on adapting these recipes to a vegetarian or vegan diet, see chapter 11, "Applications and Adaptations.")

HOMEMADE BROTH (AS AN OPTION)

Making your own broth (or even including broth in these recipes) is 100 percent optional. You may use broth out of a carton you bought at a discount store. You can just use water. It all comes down to your own preference and the time you have available. You do not need to make your own broth. However, homemade broth is certainly delicious, and I am a bit of an expert on the topic, and so I include it here for your interest.

Homemade broth caught steam on the internet beginning in about 2005 and spawned an entire industry around doing something very simple and traditional: extracting flavor and nutrition from bones. Homemade broth is a simple process that cave people likely developed. My mom learned a traditional process from a French chef in Sequoia National Park, where she waitressed as a college student in about 1965. Thanks to that chef, I grew up with broth on the stove top regularly. Forty years later, the internet and the growing whole foods movement ignited interest in this simple concept, but I noticed a good bit of strangeness in those early days.

People were seeking rather obsessively to fine-tune their broth, adding vinegar in particular to bring more minerals out of the bones. Some were making broth from whole chicken or steak, missing their chance to roast a chicken and then use the bones for a batch of broth. Further, no one seemed to notice that the bones could be used multiple

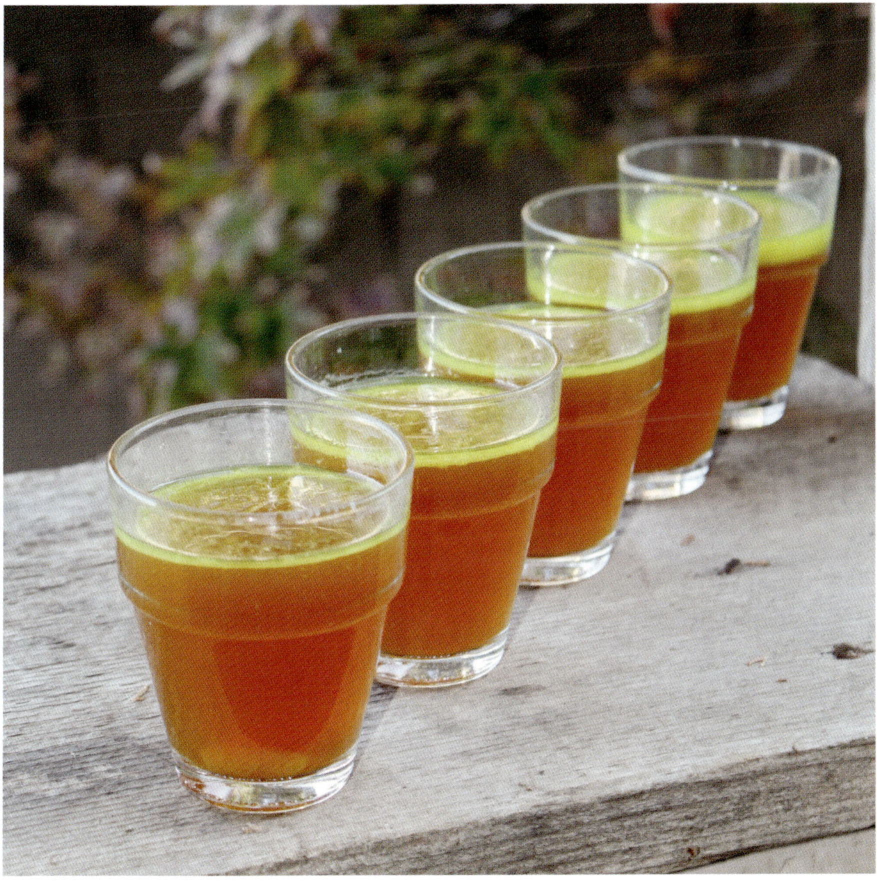

times. That French chef kept his until they fell apart completely. He kept the pot simmering, adding new bones to it every day, and removing broth from it every day. He didn't add vinegar because he didn't want vinegar in all of his recipes. Besides, the bones were falling apart anyway. The minerals in the bones were hitting that water all by themselves.

One of the big fascinations was increasing the gelatin content of broth—that gelatinous consistency similar to Jell-O. Gelatin is collagen, a nutrient many people take in powders these days, one that keeps our skin looking healthy and youthful. Bones have gelatin in them, and people were working to maximize gelatin in their broth and wondering why their homemade broth had none.

In the context of all of that emerging internet love for broth, I made a video titled "Twelve Days of Gelatin" in which I reused bones every day for twelve days, with observable gelatin in the broth each time. Rather than throwing the bones away, I just kept making new batches of broth, getting gelatin out of twelve batches. The concept took off when my friend Jenny McGruther, a nutritional therapist and herbalist, popularized it on her website Nourished Kitchen, and it became known as the continuous broth method.

All of this is to say, I was a broth expert long before I was a weight loss expert, and I offer you insight from this experience which fits like a glove with the theme of our Eat Like a Bear! observations:

- Keep it simple. Broth or stock (or whatever you want to call it) is nothing more than bones stewed in water.
- Find bones in the meat section of your supermarket or at a traditional butcher shop.
- Buy meats with bone in, cook and eat the meat portion, and then stew the bone. (Rotisserie chicken included.)
- If you really want gelatin in it, use the feet of the animal. (Yes, I know . . . and yes, you can buy animal feet.)
- Make it on days you are cooking a lot of soup and just add the fresh hot broth to your recipe. Store a quart or two of broth in the freezer.

Broth-Making: The Basic Approach

Cover bones in water. Stew for up to 24 hours. After 24 hours or so, the broth tends to get a bit bitter. Reuse the bones if it works for you.

Stew your bones any way you wish, though odor can be slightly off on the stove top. In a slow cooker, don't let a batch go for more than twenty-four hours lest it get bitter. In the pressure cooker, you can make a batch of broth in 2 to 3 hours. On long kitchen days, you can get multiple batches of broth out of that same batch of bones and pressure cooker. That would be a good day to make a large batch of soup and to put up some broth in the freezer.

Stove top: Cover bones in water. Simmer on low overnight.

Slow cooker: Cover bones in water. Simmer on low overnight.

Pressure cooker: Cover bones in water. Cook for 2 hours.

Broth-Making: Additions and Techniques

You can always step up any process to increase flavor, including broth-making. Add any or all of the following as you desire:

- Use bones with a high gelatin content: For higher gelatin content, go with the feet and knuckles. Marrow bones are excellent options as well.
- Roast the bones for additional flavor: Place the bones in a baking pan in a 350 degree oven for 30 to 45 minutes. (Longer is fine, too; this is a very forgiving step.) Cover the bones with foil to prevent the fat from splattering in your oven.
- Add a bit of vinegar: Vinegar will help draw out a bit more of the mineral content. I like vinegar in nearly everything, and so a bit of vinegar in my broth is totally fine in my opinion. Add a tablespoon or two if you choose.
- Add some vegetables: Include celery, onion, and garlic for a bit of extra flavor. Some vegetables will impart bitterness to the broth, so I advise against adding cruciferous vegetables (turnips, broccoli, cabbage, Brussels sprouts, collard greens, kale, mustard greens) and green peppers.
- Add meat: Some people add meat to the broth and end up with a richer broth, but this approach is not the most economical or flavor-enhancing use of meat, so I do not go in this direction myself.

Using and Storing the Broth

Ideally, as that broth finishes, you are working on a big pot of soup and use all or most of the broth while the broth is hot. You certainly can store the broth, but then you are taking up space in your refrigerator or freezer, and you are also reheating it later.

My usual process is to make a couple of batches of broth from one set of bones, using at least one batch for a large pot of soup, and then freeze most of the other batch by the pint (for use in some of these skillet recipes). Typically, I use a plastic freezer container with a lid to store the broth. You can add the broth to one of these recipes either frozen or semifrozen; just allow for more cook time.

PRACTICE TODAY TO SET YOUR EXPECTATIONS FOR TOMORROW

I realize that for recipes this simple you really don't need to practice because you will end up with something completely edible with no practice whatsoever. However, I encourage you to practice putting these meals together, with the aim of keeping them simple and quick so that you can get into a groove. Marvel at the simplicity and tell yourself how easy these meals will be on those very bad days.

If you use good days to practice, something important happens: through your own behavior and self-talk, you set up an expectation for yourself so that if you wake up tomorrow to a very bad day, your eating plan is in place and ready for you. You are putting your technocratic side in charge. Do not take this exercise for granted. In fact, reviewing it every day would not be too much. You need to establish a groove that you can ride every single day for a whole lot of days as you get through the grind of weight loss.

To find simple dishes for your practice, I direct you to Week 1 of the Six-Week Plan (chapter 10). For that first week, I selected what I deemed to be the most basic recipes that require minimal ingredients. In addition, you might shop for a seasoning blend such as curry, garam masala, or taco seasoning and integrate one of those blends into your make-it-quick routines, just for some extra variety. On my own bad days, my dishes look a lot like variations of the gravy dishes and panang curry dishes in this book. They are so simple that I just throw stuff in the skillet.

PREPARATION WILL REWIRE YOUR BRAIN AND SET YOUR INTENTION AS A MEAL TECHNOCRAT

Something very powerful happens when you are preparing food for tomorrow (and for next month at the same time): You are sending a strong signal to yourself about your *intention*. In the process of signaling to yourself that you *intend* to eat this way tomorrow, how much more likely are you to eat this way tomorrow? Consider the reverse: you put off planning and know in the back of your mind that you can always stop at the drive-through. Which path is the likely path to success?

Considering that part of each of us wants to be at the drive-through and eating factory-flavored fast food designed to have us clamoring for more, I would put a giant fat stack down on this: if you don't plan, you're going through that drive-through line. You could end up in that little gray area of universe two I described earlier, struggling with the proverbial potpie in your freezer.

People make comments in our social media circles all the time: "Help! I just can't help myself! I always end up caving and I just can't stop!" I believe them. If that's how they see tomorrow, then that is how tomorrow will be. They have already told me.

Let's do today and tomorrow differently from how we did yesterday. Plan for tomorrow. Start today with what you're eating. I am going to walk you through how I do it in case you need some ideas, but however you do end up working it all out is exactly what you should be doing.

Step 1: Identify Your Own Easy Favorites

Perhaps you have already done this before finding this book, but if you are just getting started with Eat Like a Bear!, I strongly encourage you to go through the Six-Week Plan in this book and then determine your three favorite easy recipes. Most people, however, first go through the recipe section and cherry-pick those they want to try, which is okay, too.

Try the easy ones. Take notes, and adjust the seasonings and such to suit yourself. Identify three easy favorites. Your three easy favorites ought to be recipes you like that also have ingredients you can find or make readily.

In my case, for instance, the fajita bowl would not be on this list because even though it is a favorite of mine, it calls for grilled fresh vegetables (which is not easy enough) and I like it with avocado (which is not always available). A better choice for me is the Zuppa Toscana because I can easily get cooked ground sausage, cauliflower, and greens.

Step 2: Become a Master in Your Own Easy Favorites

Over the next month or two, I want you to rotate these three recipes through your life with the intention of learning how to make them exactly how you like them, like a pro. Alternate them with new recipes or with your Ridiculously Big Salad for variety, as you wish, but go through these weeks working on mastering the three recipes.

Step 3: Plan Your Pantry Strategically

As you identify your easy favorites, make sure that every single day you always have something in your house for at least one of those favorite recipes. Be strategic about your pantry. Do not leave this part to chance.

By the end of Step 3, you will have stuff in your pantry and freezer that prepares you to make your favorite easy meal should you wake up tomorrow at the beginning of a bad day. If you wake up to a good day and you are inclined to try other recipes, by all means, try them. Regardless, you already know that either way, you're not rummaging through your freezer or going through the drive-through. You are ready.

Step 4: In Your New Expertise, Be Ready and Substitute Like Crazy

Here's where it all starts getting simpler and more customized to your own circumstances.

Notice how simple the recipes are in this book and that you can pretty much substitute any protein for any other, making whatever you want or bending to whatever you have on hand. That's the level of mastery you're working for.

At the risk of being obvious, the first recipe in the recipe section is Panang Chicken. That recipe could have been Panang Pork, Panang Sausage, Panang Shrimp, Panang Tofu, and so on. It could have been more or less spicy or sweet. It could have any number of vegetables under it. The recipe is completely adaptable.

Here's the process I recommend you go through, one that will help with planning and intention. By this step, you have chosen your favorite protein and have it readily available in your freezer to make one of your favorite easy meals.

Let's assume you have identified the Zuppa Toscana as your favorite, and you always keep sausage on hand. Sit down with paper and a pen and write down Zuppa Toscana. There are blank pages at the end of this book for this purpose. (You can also grab a spiral notebook from a big box store for a buck.) What else can you make easily, knowing that you have sausage on hand? Identify and write down those other simple recipes. Writing is a powerful way to set our intentions.

I sat down with a notebook and made a short list of recipes I could easily make that use the same sausage as Zuppa Toscana. Here's a snapshot of what I wrote:

Sausage

Zuppa Toscana
Sausage with gravy over green beans
Sausage, sage, Parm over zucchini
Sausage Cauliflower Teriyaki
Salsa Verde Sausage
Pesto Sausage
Kale and Sausage Soup
Sausage gravy over Konjac noodles

Notice a couple of things: there is no "Pesto Sausage" recipe in this book, nor a "Salsa Verde Sausage." I simply substituted the chicken that is in each of these recipes with sausage, creating instant favorite recipes. That's how one "easy favorite" expands to seven more and then becomes really fairly endless. You can make your version of this list.

I often keep chicken strips on hand as well. I made a similar list with my second favorite easy recipe (Panang Chicken) as the lead recipe.

Chicken Strips

Panang Chicken
Chicken Mushroom Casserole
Broccoli Chicken Skillet (or Cauliflower)
Creamy Chicken with Spinach
Salsa Verde Chicken
Pesto Chicken
Cream of Broccoli Chicken Soup

More often than not, I also have a bag of cooked shrimp in the freezer to prepare my third easy favorite, Peanut Shrimp. How might I use that shrimp for other easy meals?

Shrimp

Peanut Shrimp Skillet
Creamy Herb Shrimp
Panang Shrimp
Creamy Shrimp with Spinach
Pesto Shrimp

Pretty much any of these favorite meals I can now make in 10 minutes. The ingredients are all basics, and I almost always have ingredients on hand for any one of them. From start to finish, all of these recipes are simple, which makes them a highly competitive alternative to the drive-through. When you factor in that they are cheaper than fast food, don't make you fat, and don't weigh you down with guilt and remorse, they are setting you on a path to a much more rewarding future.

Step 5: Strategically Avoid Problematic Ingredients

I'll add a caveat that you probably already know, but it always helps to see it in writing: if there is an ingredient problematic for you in any of this, exclude it from your favorite easy recipes.

Of course, this applies to the usual issues like food intolerances, but for our purposes, I am calling out any ingredient that might make you struggle. Simply put, if you tend to overeat a particular item, you're going to have a real hard time losing weight and maintaining your weight loss if that item is an ingredient in your favorite recipes.

Cream is a common ingredient in these recipes. Let's say you love cream and can too easily overdo it. Keeping it in your refrigerator might become a problem for you. This is where adaptation and substitutions win. I will give you an example from my own life of how I manage problem food items.

First, know that I could drink a pint of cream in a day or two in my coffee if I could get away with it, but that would be nearly an extra thousand calories a day, which might as well be a "million jillion" for a short older woman like myself. If I have cream around and I start to have it in my coffee, I find myself struggling to moderate my consumption.

My rule with cream is basically this: I never put cream in my coffee at home. If my older son is home with us and he asks for cream, we buy it and I stay away from it at coffee time. The cream disappears pretty quickly and does not tend to be a big problem for me in those circumstances.

However, I allow myself cream in my coffee away from home, and that can cause another interesting problem. There are times when I spend two weeks at a time at a friend's condo on the West Coast working on projects like this book. The condo is literally right next to a grocery store: I have unlimited access to cream if I get started on it. I do not get started on it. On those trips, I cook things from this book, but I always use something other than cream in recipes that call for cream. In most recipes, you can easily substitute the cream portion with sour cream or cheese. Those substitutions are equally rich and satisfying, and more importantly, I have never had the urge to add sour cream or pepper jack cheese to my coffee. They are safer ingredients to have around.

Sure, I could try to be stronger and not drink as much cream as I am inclined to. I choose to exercise my strength by buying sour cream and pepper jack cheese, which makes life a whole lot easier.

As you go through this process, I encourage you to look at all of your foods this way. Basically, if you are eating a whole lot of something, and that something is one of the reasons you are struggling with your weight, then I would be inclined to cut it out.

chapter four

Skillet Dishes

The skillet dish started it all for us that March 2020 day at school with the Sul family, right before we all went into quarantine. Making this dish really is the most basic of all the concepts in this book. This simple technique is highly adaptable to flavors and ingredients.

People ask me all the time about recipe specifics; they worry that they are doing it wrong. Let's get right to it and make sure you're not doing it wrong:

- If you feel compelled to use only fresh vegetables and spend your time dicing, slicing, mincing, and julienning them instead of practicing the technique of grabbing a bag of inexpensive, frozen vegetables right out of your freezer, ripping the bag open, and dumping them in a skillet or pot, then you very well could be doing it wrong.
- If you get concerned because your broth is coming out of a carton or because you do not see enough gelatin in your homemade broth, then you very well could be doing it wrong.
- If you are worried that you really should have used ground turkey instead of ground chicken, then you very well could be doing it wrong.
- If you're worried that you don't have onion powder or that you are allergic to it and, therefore, can't make recipes that use onion powder or can't use this framework in general, then you very well might be doing it wrong.

What you are really doing here is taking a very simple meal approach that is highly effective for weight loss and learning how to make the meal preparation second nature. In a year from now if you've forgotten all of these recipes and do not even consult the book because you are just throwing stuff together in your kitchen, consider that a complete success, especially if this whole process has helped you live the life you want to live.

This technique is utterly adaptable. If your favorite flavor or protein and vegetable combination is not in this book, all you need to do is follow the framework using your preferred ingredients. I hear it in the community all the time: "Isn't it something when you've really learned it and you can adapt it to *anything*?" It sure is. It becomes etched in your brain somewhere at some point, but that etching happens on your good days.

THE BASIC SKILLET PROCESS

This is a highly formulaic and simple meal type. Each recipe is organized in the same way with the amount of cooking oil given first, followed by the main protein and the vegetables, and then a list of ingredients for the sauce. Some recipes have additional ingredients added at the end, often a dairy item.

You can make these dishes more "gourmet" by, for example, mincing fresh garlic—or just follow these very simple steps.

MAKE IT A DOUBLE?

Scale any of these recipes into the sky. Except for a couple of soups, I have never more than doubled the recipes here, but there is no reason not to. They are all fairly lightly seasoned, so pop it all together and taste-test the final batch for flavor.

In my household, I often double these recipes and eat about half myself for my one ridiculous meal. Then my husband and two boys split the rest. They each eat two to three meals a day, so they would not likely eat a giant portion with me.

On occasion, I double the recipe and stash a portion in the freezer for a later date, a "just in case" moment. These meals are so easy to make that I don't tend to lean on freezing the cooked meals, but they certainly are convenient.

Step 1: Warm Your Skillet and Oil

Warm your skillet on medium high and heat the oil.

Step 2: Gather Your Vegetables and Dump Them In

Gather the vegetable base portion of the recipe (often frozen broccoli or cauliflower) and add it to the skillet.

Step 3: Add Your Protein

Especially if the protein is frozen, add it on top of the vegetables so that it can begin to defrost. Cover the skillet with a lid as you mix up the sauce.

Step 4: Mix Up the Sauce and Add It

The ingredients for the sauce are listed below the main protein and vegetables, just above the recipe note that says "Cook, then add." It typically includes broth and seasonings.

Make your sauce by mixing the seasonings in with the broth, and stir them together well before adding to the skillet. In this step, include any extras for the sauce, such as tomato paste or peanut powder. Stir in a thickener at this stage if you choose—glucomannan powder or xanthan gum are the best options. Add the sauce to the skillet. Cover.

Your cook time will vary based on your stove, elevation, and ingredients. Whole frozen cauliflower florets will take a good bit longer to cook than frozen cauliflower rice. Adding frozen protein to the skillet will increase the cooking time as well. For a dish with larger florets and with a frozen protein item, allow about 20 minutes and use a fork to check for doneness. For smaller items such as cauliflower rice or greens beans, check at the 10-minute point.

Step 5: When Cooked, Add the Other Stuff

Once cooked, add ingredients in the lower part of the recipe, stirring in items such as cream. Cheese and garnishes can be sprinkled on top or mixed in, as you desire. Adjust for salt and pepper.

The cream and cheese items are added at this final stage to avoid curdling. If you add them in the first step (which you can do) and they do curdle, no worries: the dish is still edible.

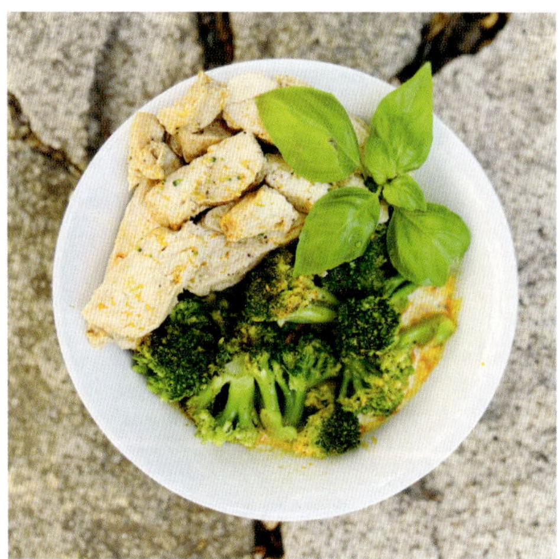

Panang Chicken

1 tablespoon (15 ml) cooking oil
8 ounces (225 g) chicken breast, cooked
12 ounces (340 g) frosen broccoli
½ cup (120 ml) chicken broth
1 cup (240 ml) coconut cream
½ teaspoon (2 g) garlic powder
½ teaspoon (1 g) onion powder
½ teaspoon (3 g) salt
½ teaspoon (1 g) pepper
¼ teaspoon (½ g) ginger powder
½ teaspoon (1 g) ground coriander
½ teaspoon (1 g) ground cumin
¼ teaspoon (1 g) turmeric
⅛ teaspoon (¼ g) cayenne
⅛ teaspoon (½ g) annatto, optional
Sweetener to taste, optional
(*1,070 calories, 24 grams net carbs*)

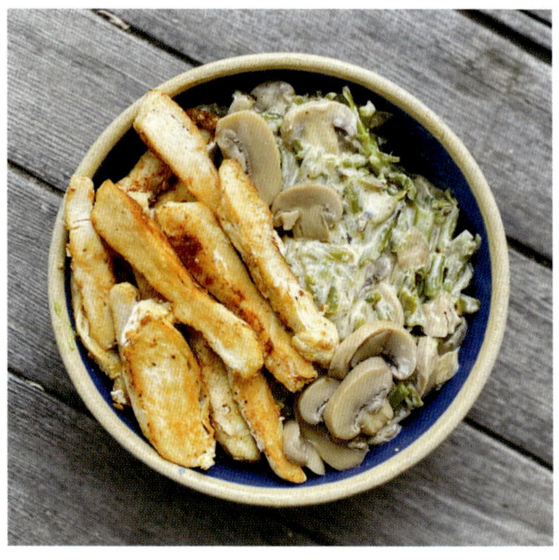

Chicken Mushroom Casserole

2 tablespoons (30 ml) cooking oil
8 ounces (225 g) chicken breast, cooked
12 ounces (340 g) frozen green beans
4 ounces (115 g) canned mushrooms, drained
½ cup (120 ml) chicken broth
½ teaspoon (2 g) garlic powder
½ teaspoon (1 g) onion powder
½ teaspoon (3 g) salt
½ teaspoon (1 g) pepper

Cook, then add:
½ cup (120 ml) cream
(*1,175 calories, 24 grams net carbs*)

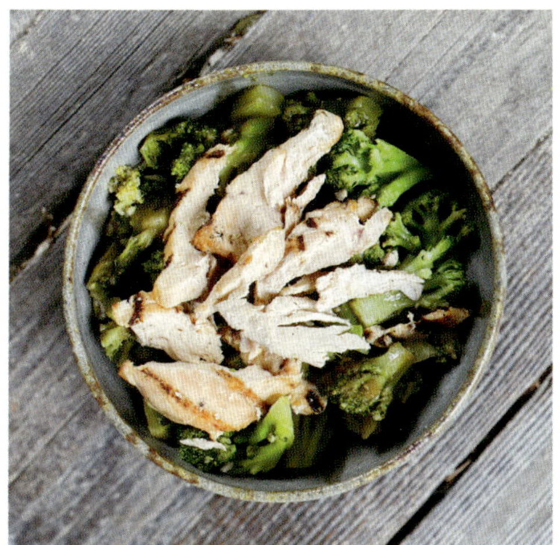

Chicken Teriyaki

2 tablespoons (30 ml) cooking oil
8 ounces (225 g) chicken breast, cooked
12 ounces (340 g) broccoli, frozen
½ cup (120 ml) chicken broth
2 tablespoons (30 ml) soy sauce/tamari
½ teaspoon (2 g) garlic powder
½ teaspoon (1 g) onion powder
½ teaspoon (3 g) salt
½ teaspoon (1 g) pepper

Cook, then add:

¼ cup (30 g) peanuts
(*1,053 calories, 23 grams net carbs*)

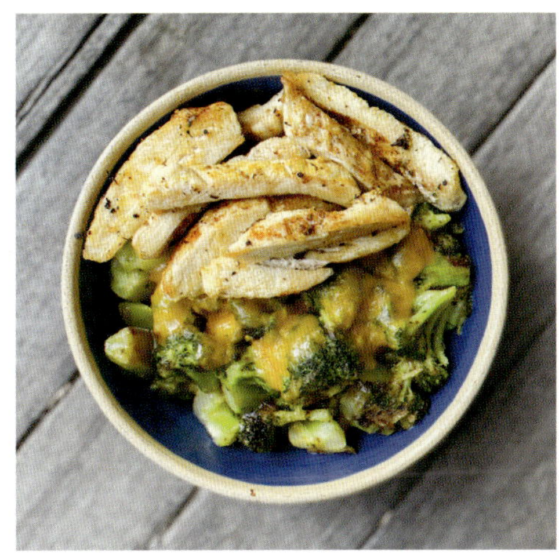

Broccoli Chicken Skillet

1 tablespoon (15 ml) cooking oil
8 ounces (225 g) chicken, cooked
12 ounces (340 g) frozen broccoli
½ cup (120 ml) chicken broth
½ teaspoon (2 g) garlic powder
½ teaspoon (1 g) onion powder
½ teaspoon (3 g) salt
½ teaspoon (1 g) pepper

Cook, then add:

½ cup (50 g) grated Cheddar
(*1,070 calories, 19 grams net carbs*)

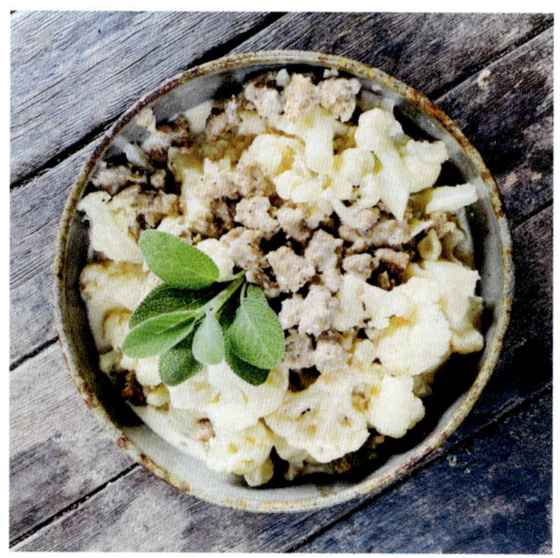

Sausage and Mushroom Gravy

1 tablespoon (15 ml) cooking oil
8 ounces (225 g) ground sausage, cooked
12 ounces (340 g) frozen cauliflower
4 ounces (115 g) canned mushrooms, drained
½ cup (120 ml) chicken broth
½ teaspoon (2 g) garlic powder
½ teaspoon (1 g) onion powder
½ teaspoon (3 g) salt
½ teaspoon (1 g) pepper

Cook, then add:

¼ cup (60 ml) cream
(*1,154 calories, 18 grams net carbs*)

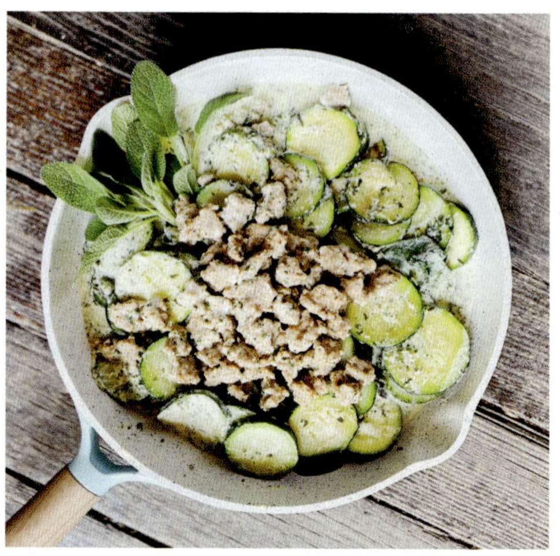

Sausage and Sage

1 tablespoon (15 ml) cooking oil
8 ounces (225 g) ground sausage, cooked
12 ounces (340 g) frozen zucchini
½ cup (120 ml) chicken broth
2 tablespoons (3 ml) dried parsley
20 sage leaves
½ teaspoon (2 g) garlic powder
½ teaspoon (1 g) onion powder
½ teaspoon (3 g) salt
½ teaspoon (1 g) pepper

Cook, then add:

½ cup (120 g) ricotta
¼ cup (30 g) grated Parmesan
(*1,185 calories, 13 grams net carbs*)

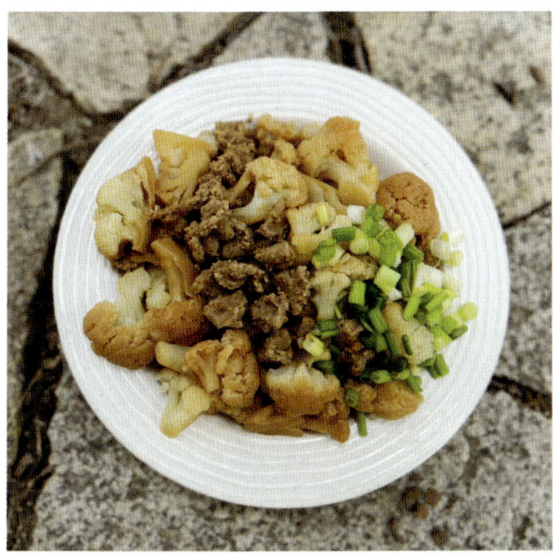

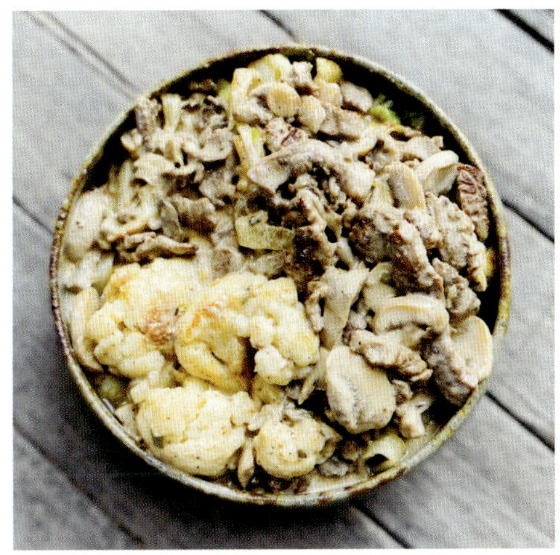

Sausage Cauliflower Teriyaki

3 tablespoons (45 ml) cooking oil
8 ounces (225 g) sausage, cooked
12 ounces (340 g) frozen cauliflower
½ cup (120 ml) chicken broth
2 tablespoons (30 ml) soy sauce/tamari
1 teaspoon (5 ml) sesame oil
½ teaspoon (2 g) garlic powder
½ teaspoon (1 g) ginger powder
½ teaspoon (1 g) pepper
Sweetener to taste, optional
(*864 calories, 14 grams net carbs*)

Beef Stroganoff

1 tablespoon (15 ml) cooking oil
8 ounces (225 g) beef strips (or ground beef), cooked
12 ounces (340 g) frozen cauliflower
4 ounces (115 g) canned mushrooms, drained
½ cup (120 ml) beef broth
1 tablespoon (2 g) dried parsley
½ teaspoon (2 g) garlic powder
½ teaspoon (1 g) onion powder
½ teaspoon (3 g) salt
½ teaspoon (1 g) pepper
½ teaspoon (1 g) paprika
1 tablespoon (15 ml) vinegar

Cook, then add:

½ cup (120 ml) sour cream
(*1,050 calories, 17 grams net carbs*)

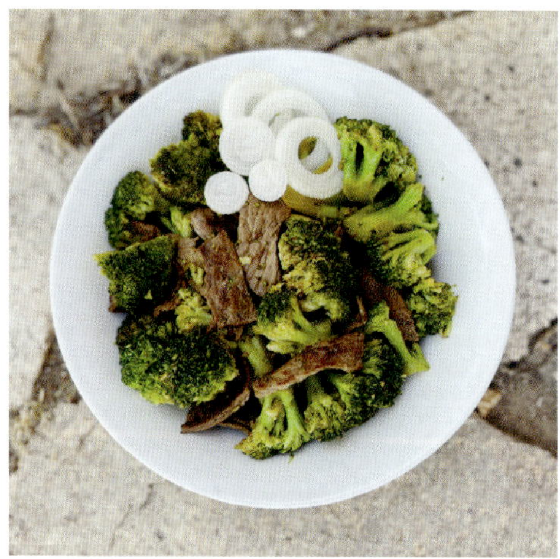

Beef Teriyaki

2 tablespoons (30 ml) cooking oil
8 ounces (225 g) beef, cooked
12 ounces (340 g) frozen broccoli
½ cup (120 ml) beef broth
2 tablespoons (30 ml) soy sauce/tamari
1 teaspoon (5 ml) sesame oil
½ teaspoon (2 g) garlic powder
1 teaspoon (2 g) ginger powder
½ teaspoon (1 g) pepper
Sweetener to taste, optional
(*1,000 calories, 18 grams net carbs*)

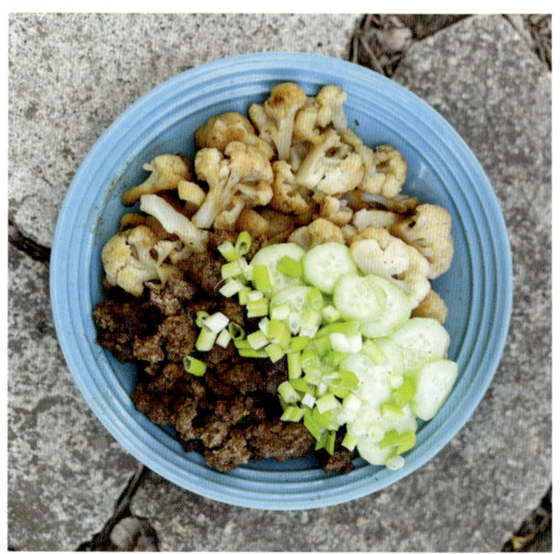

Korean Beef

2 tablespoons (30 ml) cooking oil
8 ounces (225 g) beef, cooked
12 ounces (340 g) frozen cauliflower
½ cup (120 ml) beef broth
2 tablespoons (30 ml) soy sauce/tamari
1 teaspoon (5 ml) sesame oil
½ teaspoon (2 g) garlic powder
½ teaspoon (1 g) ginger powder
½ teaspoon (1 g) pepper
⅛ teaspoon (¼ g) cayenne

Cook, then add:
Green onions and sliced cucumber, optional
(*990 calories, 14 grams net carbs*)

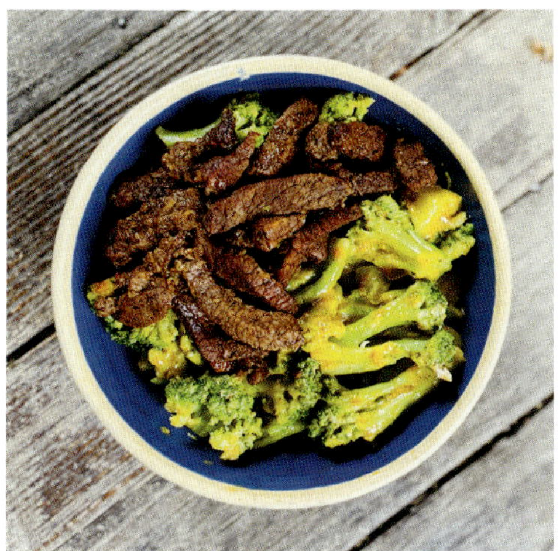

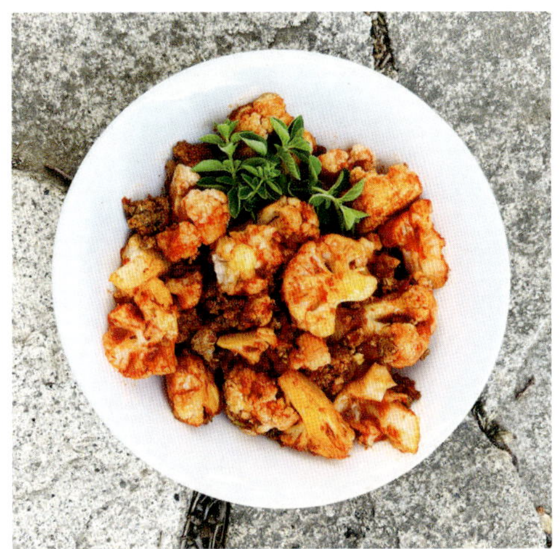

Panang Beef

1 tablespoon (15 ml) cooking oil
8 ounces (225 g) beef, cooked
12 ounces (340 g) frozen broccoli
½ cup (120 ml) beef broth
½ cup (120 ml) coconut cream
½ teaspoon (2 g) garlic powder
½ teaspoon (1 g) onion powder
½ teaspoon (3 g) salt
½ teaspoon (1 g) pepper
½ teaspoon (1 g) ginger powder
½ teaspoon (1 g) ground coriander
½ teaspoon (1 g) ground cumin
¼ teaspoon (1 g) turmeric
⅛ teaspoon (¼ g) cayenne
⅛ teaspoon (½ g) annatto, optional
Sweetener to taste, optional
(*1,070 calories, 21 grams net carbs*)

Cajun Garlic Beef

2 tablespoons (30 ml) cooking oil
8 ounces (225 g) beef, cooked
12 ounces (340 g) frozen cauliflower
½ cup (120 ml) beef broth
1 tablespoon (15 ml) tomato paste
1 teaspoon (3 g) paprika
½ teaspoon (2 g) garlic powder
½ teaspoon (1 g) onion powder
½ teaspoon (3 g) salt
½ teaspoon (2 g) pepper
⅛ teaspoon (1 g) cayenne
½ teaspoon (1 g) ground oregano
¼ teaspoon (½ g) ground thyme
(*950 calories, 13 grams net carbs*)

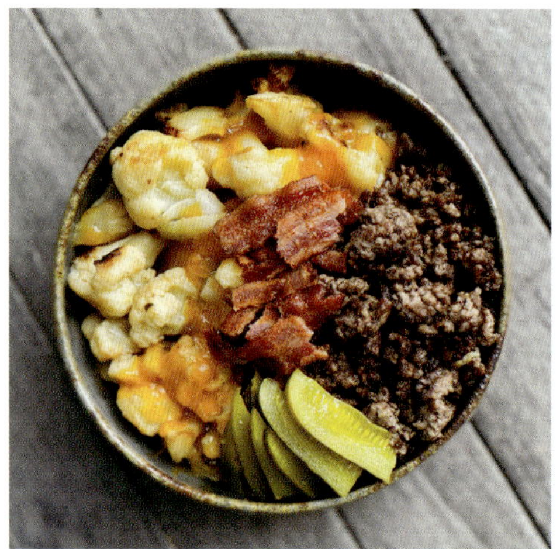

Cheeseburger in a Bowl

1 tablespoon (15 ml) cooking oil
8 ounces (225 g) ground beef, cooked
12 ounces (340 g) frozen cauliflower
½ cup (120 ml) beef broth
½ teaspoon (2 g) garlic powder
½ teaspoon (1 g) onion powder
½ teaspoon (3 g) salt
½ teaspoon (1 g) pepper
Cook, then add:
¼ cup (25 g) grated Cheddar
1 pickle spear, sliced
½ white onion, thinly sliced
2 slices of bacon, chopped

Cheeseburger salad dressing (or sour cream seasoned with garlic):

2 tablespoons (30 ml) mayonnaise
2 tablespoons (30 ml) Greek yogurt
Dash of paprika
1 tablespoon (15 ml) dill pickle juice
½ teaspoon (2 g) prepared mustard
½ teaspoon (2 g) apple cider vinegar
Sweetener to taste, optional

(*1,300 calories, 21 grams net carbs*)

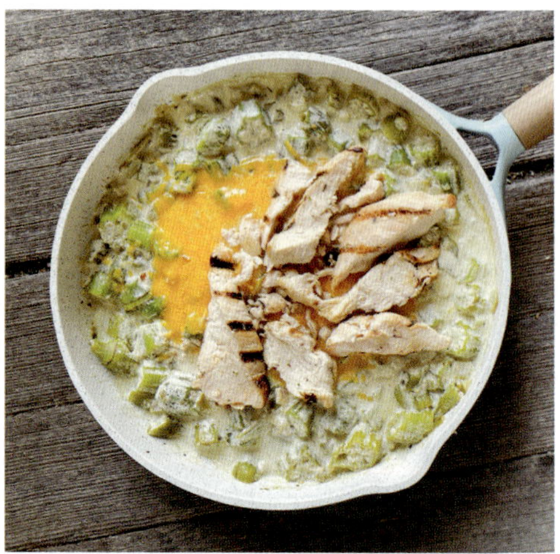

Salsa Verde Chicken

1 tablespoon (15 ml) cooking oil
8 ounces (225 g) chicken breast, cooked
12 ounces (340 g) frozen okra
½ cup (120 ml) chicken broth
¾ cup (180 ml) salsa verde
1 teaspoon (3 g) ground cumin
½ teaspoon (1 g) ground coriander
½ teaspoon (3 g) salt
½ teaspoon (1 g) pepper

Cook, then add:

½ cup (120 ml) full-fat sour cream
¼ cup (25 g) grated Cheddar

(*1,213 calories, 33 grams net carbs*)

chapter five

Sautés

If these recipes seem awfully similar to the skillet dishes, they are. In fact, the only difference is the amount of liquid and a slight difference in the process. The skillet dishes use more liquid and allow you to walk away from the skillet while the food is cooking. The skillet dishes and the soup dishes are absolutely the easiest recipes in this book. You put all of the stuff in the skillet, set a timer, and walk away for a bit. However, you will likely end up bored with the texture of basically a boiled vegetable. This sauté approach requires a bit more tending but will give you some variation in texture.

THE BASIC SAUTÉ PROCESS

Here's your basic process: Warm your skillet on high and add a touch of cooking oil. Add your primary vegetable to skillet. At this point, if I have a skillet full of large frozen vegetables (such as cauliflower florets), I turn the heat to medium and put a lid on the skillet for about 10 minutes to allow the vegetables to defrost. Then I remove the lid and finish cooking them on high heat, browning them a bit in most cases. This is the stage you will tend the dish so that you do not burn the vegetables.

Simultaneously, I put a second skillet on medium low and defrost the protein item separately. Keep a lid on this skillet and add a bit of water to keep the item from drying out.

Once the protein is heated through, add it to the vegetables. Make your sauce by mixing the seasonings in with the broth, and stir them together well before adding to the skillet. In this step, include any extras for the sauce, such as tomato paste or peanut powder. In the final 5 minutes or so, add the sauce or seasoning mix to the skillet with the vegetables and meat, taking care to sprinkle or pour the seasonings across them.

Once cooked, add ingredients in the lower part of the recipe, stirring in items such as cream. Cheese and garnishes can be sprinkled on top or mixed in, as you desire. Adjust for salt and pepper.

Note: All the following recipes are for a single serving and should constitute your single meal or total caloric intake for the day.

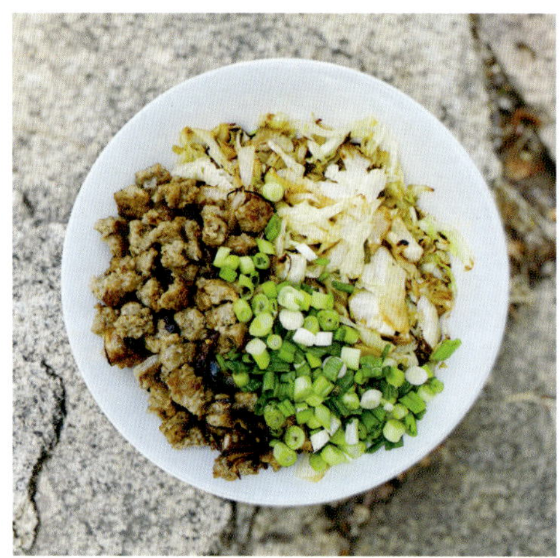

Eggroll in a Bowl

2 tablespoons (30 ml) cooking oil
8 ounces (225 g) ground sausage, cooked
½ head cabbage, sliced
½ teaspoon (2 g) garlic powder
½ teaspoon (1 g) ginger powder
½ teaspoon (1 g) pepper
2 tablespoons (30 ml) soy sauce/tamari

Cook, then add:

3 green onions, sliced
(*1,080 calories, 19 grams net carbs*)

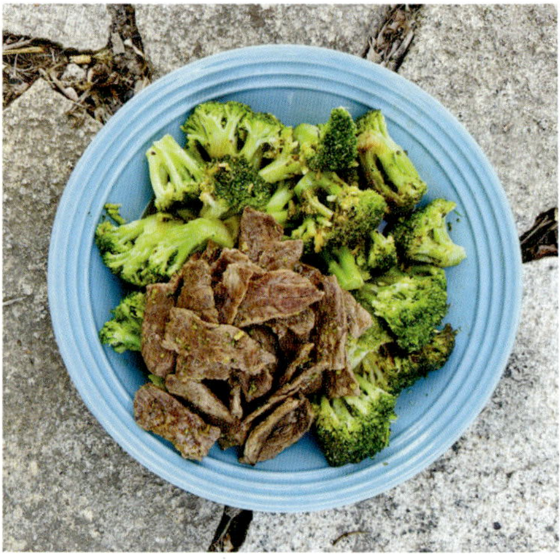

Broccoli Beef Stir-Fry

1 tablespoon (15 ml) cooking oil
8 ounces (225 g) beef, cooked
12 ounces (340 g) frozen broccoli
¼ cup (60 ml) beef broth
2 tablespoons (30 ml) soy sauce/tamari
1 tablespoon (15 ml) apple cider vinegar
½ teaspoon (2 g) garlic powder
½ teaspoon (1 g) ginger powder
½ teaspoon (1 g) pepper
⅛ teaspoon (¼ g) cayenne
(*920 calories, 22 grams net carbs*)

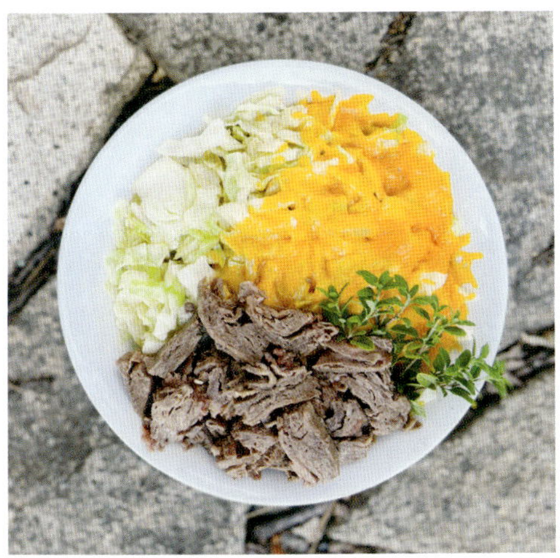

Cheesy Cabbage Stir-Fry

1 teaspoon (5 g) cooking oil
8 ounces (225 g) beef strips, cooked
½ head cabbage, chopped
¼ cup (60 ml) beef broth
½ teaspoon (2 g) garlic powder
½ teaspoon (1 g) onion powder
½ teaspoon (3 g) salt
½ teaspoon (1 g) pepper
½ teaspoon (1 g) paprika

Cook, then add:

½ cup (50 g) grated Cheddar
(*1,210 calories, 22 grams net carbs*)

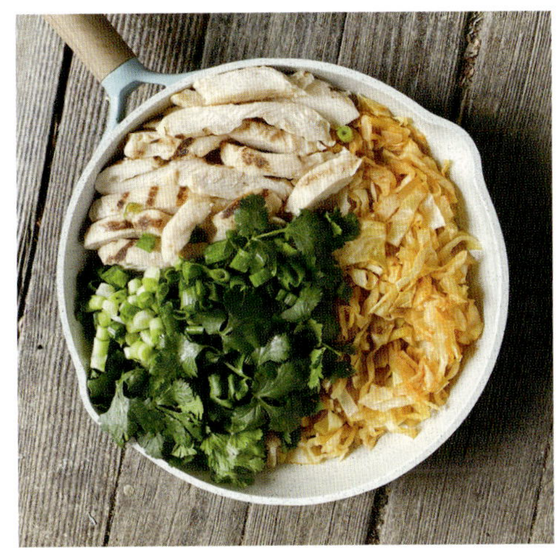

Peanut Pork Stir-Fry

3 tablespoons (45 ml) cooking oil
8 ounces (225 g) pork (strips or sausage), cooked
½ head cabbage, chopped
¼ cup (60 ml) chicken broth
2 tablespoons (30 ml) soy sauce/tamari
1 teaspoon (5 ml) sesame oil
3 tablespoons (18 g) peanut powder
½ teaspoon (2 g) garlic powder
½ teaspoon (1 g) ginger powder
½ teaspoon (1 g) pepper

Cook, then add:

3 green onions, sliced
(*1,050 calories, 22 grams net carbs*)

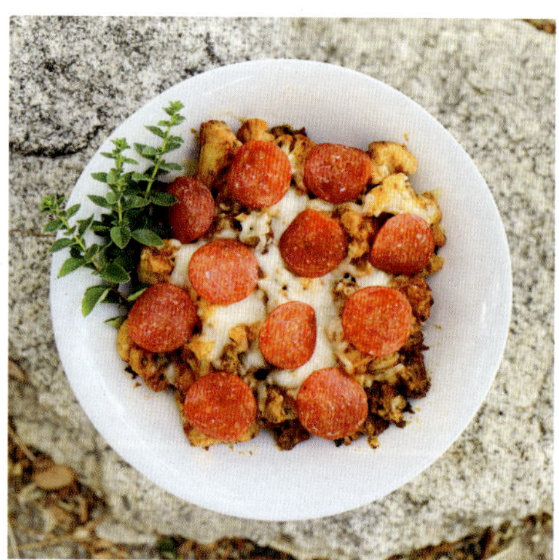

Pizza in a Bowl

2 tablespoons (30 ml) cooking oil
3 ounces (90 g) pepperoni
5 ounces (140 g) Italian sausage, cooked
12 ounces (340 g) frozen cauliflower
½ cup (120 ml) beef broth
2 tablespoons (30 ml) tomato paste
1 tablespoon (5 g) ground basil
1 tablespoon (5 g) ground oregano
1 teaspoon (1 g) ground thyme
½ teaspoon (2 g) garlic powder
½ teaspoon (1 g) onion powder
½ teaspoon (3 g) salt
½ teaspoon (1 g) pepper

Cook, then add:

½ cup (50 g) grated mozzarella cheese
(*1,080 calories, 18 grams net carbs*)

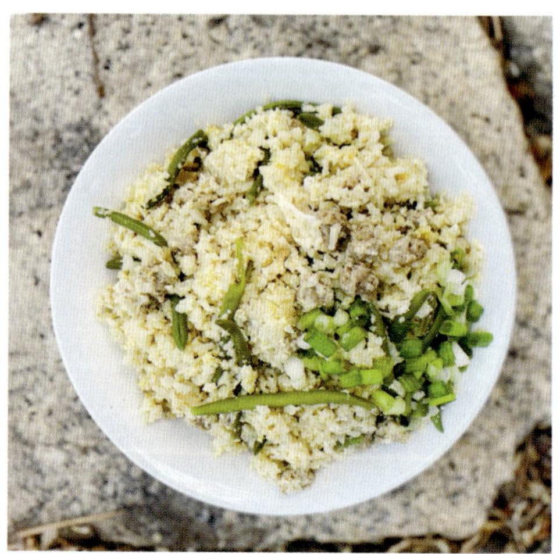

Pork Faux Rice

2 tablespoons (30 ml) cooking oil
4 ounces (115 g) sausage, cooked
10 ounces (300 g) frozen cauliflower rice
4 ounces (115 g) frozen green beans
¼ cup (60 ml) chicken broth
2 tablespoons (30 ml) soy sauce/tamari
½ teaspoon (2 g) garlic powder
½ teaspoon (1 g) onion powder
½ teaspoon (1 g) pepper
½ teaspoon (1 g) ginger powder

Cook, then add:

2 eggs, beaten and stirred in at the end of cooking
4 green onions, sliced
(*900 calories, 18 grams net carbs*)

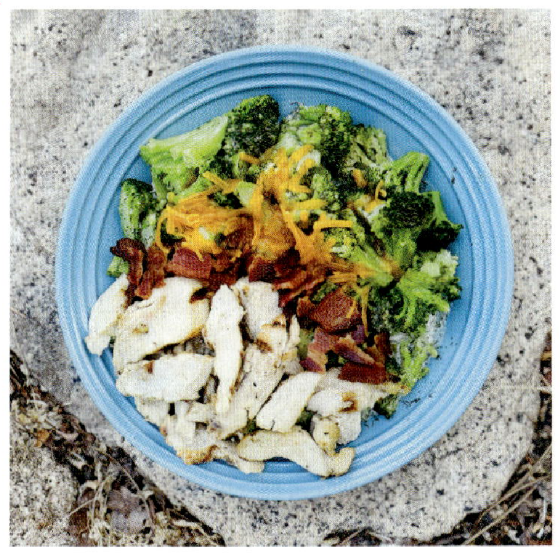

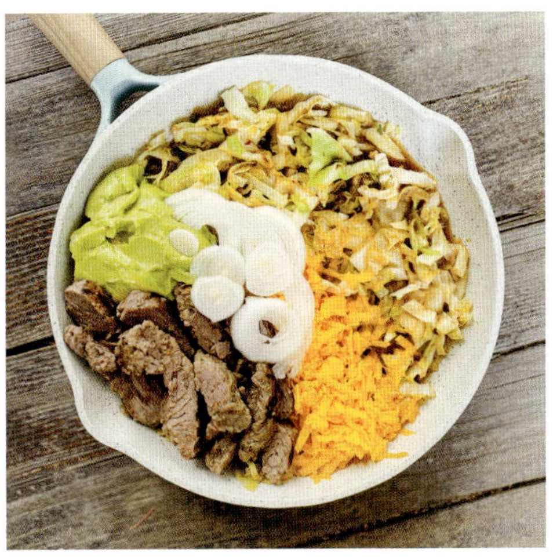

Chicken Bacon Ranch

1 tablespoon (15 ml) cooking oil
6 ounces (180 g) chicken breast, cooked
12 ounces (340 g) frozen broccoli
¼ cup (60 ml) chicken broth
½ teaspoon (2 g) garlic powder
½ teaspoon (1 g) onion powder
½ teaspoon (2 g) salt
½ teaspoon (1 g) pepper
1 tablespoon (2 g) dried parsley
1 tablespoon (3 g) dried dill

Cook, then add:

¼ cup (60 ml) cream
½ cup (50 g) grated Cheddar
4 slices crisp bacon, chopped
(*1,120 calories, 19 grams net carbs*)

Taco in a Bowl

1 teaspoon (5 ml) cooking oil
8 ounces (225 g) beef strips, cooked
½ head cabbage, chopped
¼ cup (60 ml) beef broth
½ teaspoon (2 g) garlic powder
½ teaspoon (1 g) onion powder
½ teaspoon (3 g) salt
½ teaspoon (1 g) pepper
1 teaspoon (3 g) chili powder
1 teaspoon (2 g) ground cumin
½ teaspoon (1 g) ground oregano

Cook, then add:

½ cup (50 g) grated Cheddar
½ white onion, thinly sliced
Small avocado, sliced
(*1,240 calories, 26 grams net carbs*)

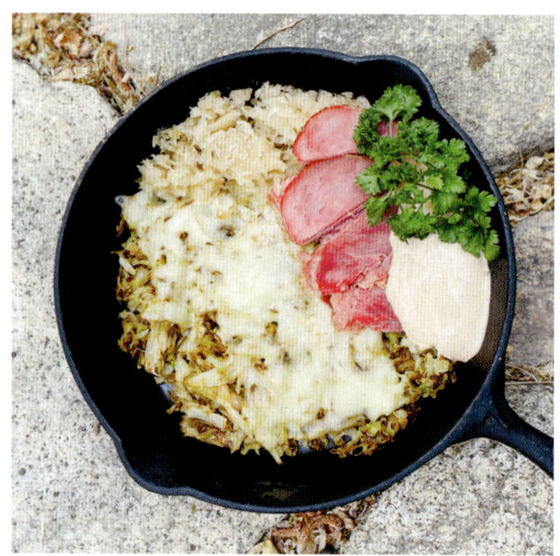

Reuben in a Bowl

1 tablespoon (15 ml) cooking oil
8 ounces (225 g) corned beef, cooked
½ head cabbage, sliced
¼ cup (60 ml) beef broth
½ teaspoon (2 g) garlic powder
½ teaspoon (1 g) onion powder
½ teaspoon (3 g) salt
½ teaspoon (1 g) pepper

Cook, then melt:

2 slices Swiss cheese

Then add the Russian dressing:

2 tablespoons (30 ml) mayonnaise
2 tablespoons (30 ml) Greek yogurt
1 tablespoon (15 ml) ketchup (no sugar added)
½ teaspoon (2 ml) horseradish
⅛ teaspoon (¼ g) cayenne
¼ teaspoon (½ g) paprika
(*1,170 calories, 21 grams net carbs*)

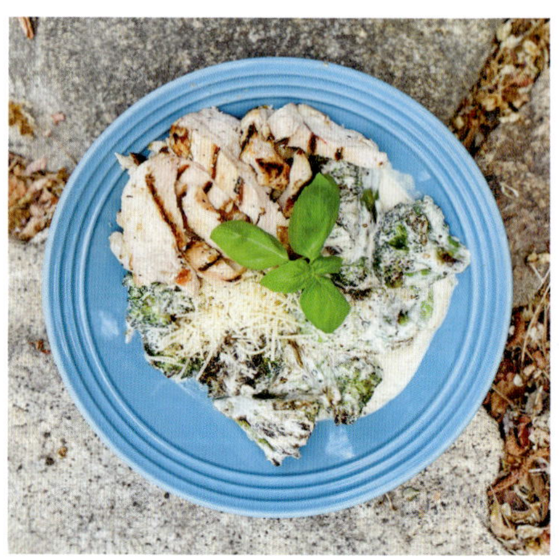

Chicken Alfredo

1 tablespoon (15 ml) cooking oil
8 ounces (225 g) chicken strips, cooked
12 ounces (340 g) frozen broccoli
½ cup (120 ml) chicken broth
½ teaspoon (2 g) garlic powder
½ teaspoon (1 g) onion powder
½ teaspoon (3 g) salt
½ teaspoon (1 g) pepper

Cook, then add:

½ cup (120 ml) cream
¼ cup (30 g) grated Parmesan
(1,140 calories, 22 grams net carbs)

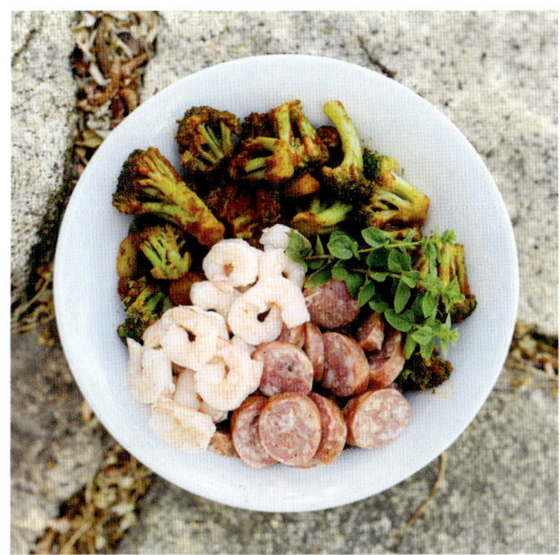

Jambalaya

2 tablespoons (30 ml) cooking oil
4 ounces (115 g) sausage, cooked
12 ounces (340 g) frozen broccoli
½ cup (120 ml) chicken broth
2 tablespoons (30 ml) tomato paste
½ teaspoon (2 g) garlic powder
½ teaspoon (1 g) onion powder
½ teaspoon (3 g) salt
½ teaspoon (1 g) pepper
½ teaspoon (1 g) paprika
½ teaspoon (1 g) ground oregano
½ teaspoon (1 g) ground thyme
⅛ teaspoon (¼ g) ground cayenne

Cook, then add:

4 ounces (115 g) shrimp, cooked
(*640 calories, 24 grams net carbs*)

VARIATION: STIR-FRY WITH GRILLED VEGETABLES

These dishes simply add grilled vegetables to the finished dish. Grill the onions and peppers in a separate skillet, on high in a bit of cooking oil. Grill them until they are caramelized. This step takes a bit more time, but the flavor is well worth it if you have the time and inclination.

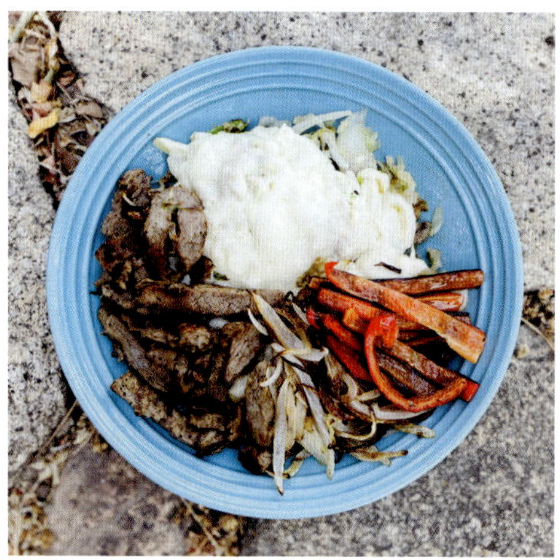

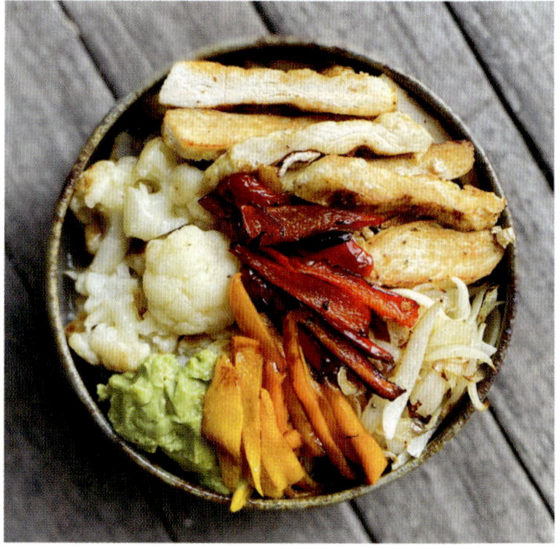

Philly Cheesesteak in a Bowl

1 tablespoon (15 ml) cooking oil
8 ounces (225 g) steak strips, cooked
12 ounces (340 g) cabbage, chopped
¼ cup (60 ml) beef broth
½ teaspoon (2 g) garlic powder
½ teaspoon (1 g) onion powder
½ teaspoon (3 g) salt
½ teaspoon (1 g) pepper

Cook, then add:

3 slices provolone

Separately:

Grill ½ white onion, ½ bell pepper in 1 tablespoon (15 ml) cooking oil, add to skillet.

(*1,240 calories, 23 grams net carbs*)

Chicken Fajita Stir-Fry

1 tablespoon (15 ml) cooking oil
8 ounces (225 g) chicken, cooked
12 ounces (340 g) frozen cauliflower
¼ cup (60 ml) chicken broth
½ teaspoon (2 g) garlic powder
½ teaspoon (1 g) onion powder
½ teaspoon (3 g) salt
½ teaspoon (1 g) pepper
1 teaspoon (3 g) chili powder
1 teaspoon (2 g) ground cumin
½ teaspoon (1 g) ground oregano

Cook, then add:

½ cup (120 ml) guacamole (on the side)

Separately:

Grill ½ white onion, ½ bell pepper in 3 tablespoons (45 ml) cooking oil, add to skillet.

(*1,170 calories, 18 grams net carbs*)

chapter six

Soup

You know all those ridiculously simple skillet recipes you just read about in the previous chapter? Are you excited to apply more of that same simple? Then you have come to the exact right chapter, because this collection of recipes is pretty much the exact same as the skillet section; they simply have more broth. That's it.

Do you see why some of my gourmet friends think I am now an embarrassment to the world of cooking? Yes, this is exactly why. May we all get trim behind this embarrassment.

In fact, you can turn any of these soup recipes into skillet dishes by using about ½ cup of broth instead of 2 cups. Turn any of the skillet dishes into soups by using 2 cups of broth instead of ½ cup. Voilà!

THE BASIC SOUP PROCESS

This is a highly formulaic and simple meal type. Make it more gourmet or follow these very simple steps.

Step 1: Warm Your Skillet and Oil

Warm your skillet on medium high.

Step 2: Gather Your Ingredients and Dump Them In

For each of the recipes below, gather all ingredients in the top portion of the recipe (all of those above the line "Cook, then add").

Combine the main vegetable and meat ingredients in your warming skillet. (Of course, if you didn't prewarm your skillet, turn it on now.)

Step 3: Mix Up the Sauce and Add It

Make your sauce by mixing the seasonings in a bowl with the broth: stir them together well before adding to the skillet. In this step, Include any extras for the sauce, such as tomato paste or peanut powder. Add a thickener at this stage if you choose—glucomannan powder or xanthan gum are the best options. Add the sauce to the skillet. Cover.

As with the skillet dishes, the soup dishes will take 10 to 20 minutes to cook. They could take a few minutes longer, depending on how large your vegetables are and how soft you like them. Check them for doneness with a fork and make a note of the cook time.

Step 4: When Cooked, Add the Other Stuff

Once cooked, add ingredients in the lower part of the recipe, stirring in items such as cream. Cheese and garnishes can be sprinkled on top or mixed in, as you desire. Adjust for salt and pepper.

The cream and cheese items are added at this final stage to avoid curdling. If you add them in the first step (which you can do) and they do curdle, no worries: the dish is still edible.

Note: All the following recipes are for a single serving and should constitute your single meal or total caloric intake for the day.

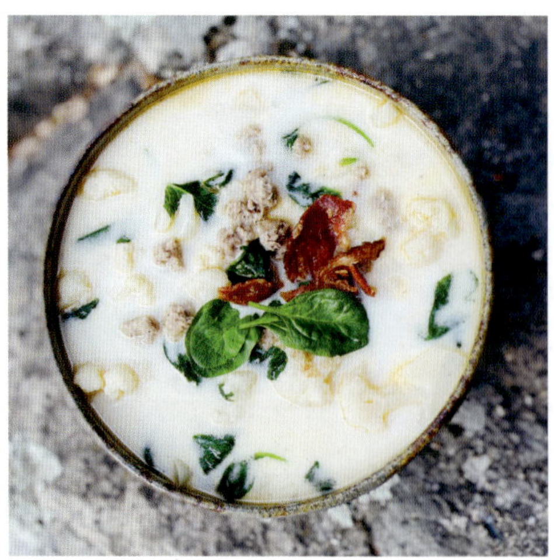

Zuppa Toscana Soup

8 ounces (225 g) ground sausage, cooked
12 ounces (340 g) frozen cauliflower
1 quart (1 liter) beef broth
1 cup (30 g) raw spinach
½ teaspoon (2 g) garlic powder
½ teaspoon (1 g) onion powder
½ teaspoon (3 g) salt
½ teaspoon (1 g) pepper

Cook, then add:

¼ cup (60 ml) cream
4 slices crisp bacon, optional
(*1,032 calories, 12 grams net carbs*)

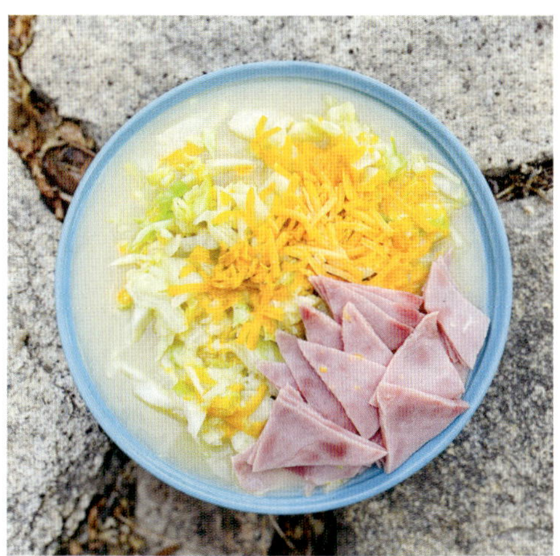

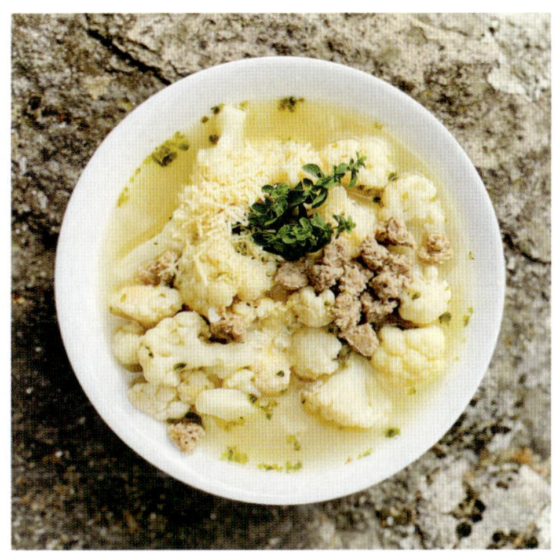

Ham and Cheese Soup

8 ounces (225 g) ham, cooked
½ head cabbage, chopped
1 quart (1 liter) chicken broth
½ teaspoon (2 g) garlic powder
½ teaspoon (1 g) onion powder
½ teaspoon (3 g) salt
½ teaspoon (1 g) pepper

Cook, then add:

1 cup (100 g) grated Cheddar
(*1,000 calories, 23 grams net carbs*)

Parmesan Herb Sausage Soup

8 ounces (225 g) sausage, cooked
12 ounces (340 g) frozen cauliflower
1 quart (1 liter) chicken broth
½ teaspoon (2 g) garlic powder
½ teaspoon (1 g) onion powder
½ teaspoon (3 g) salt
½ teaspoon (1 g) pepper
2 teaspoons (4 g) ground oregano or parsley

Cook, then add:

½ cup (60 g) grated Parmesan
(*1,060 calories, 17 grams net carbs*)

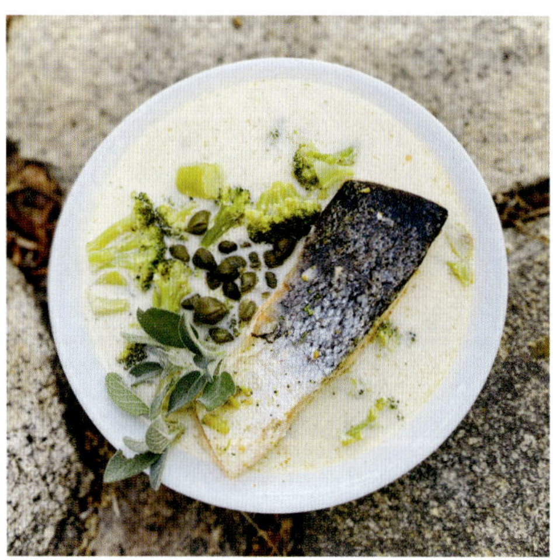

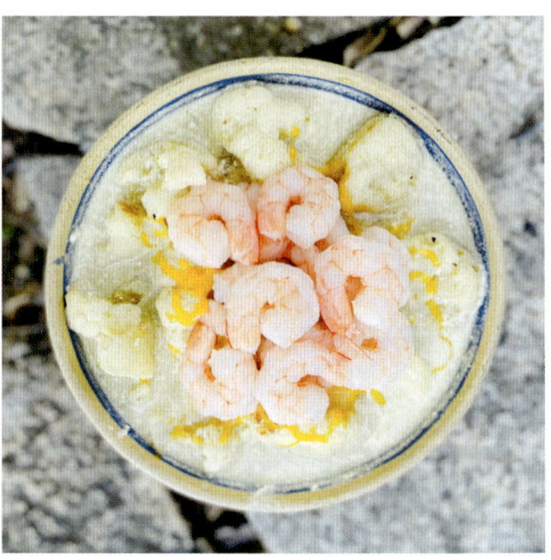

Creamy Salmon with Capers

8 ounces (225 g) frozen salmon or white fish (Use the "frozen fish" process on page 88.)

12 ounces (340 g) frozen broccoli

3 cups (710 ml) chicken broth

1 tablespoon (15 ml) Dijon mustard

½ teaspoon (2 g) garlic powder

½ teaspoon (1 g) onion powder

½ teaspoon (3 g) salt

½ teaspoon (1 g) pepper

Cook then add:

2 tablespoons (15 g) capers, optional

½ cup (120 ml) cream

(*1,000 calories, 23 grams net carbs*)

Salsa Verde Shrimp

12 ounces (340 g) frozen cauliflower

2 cups (470 ml) chicken broth

¾ cup (180 ml) salsa verde

1 teaspoon (2 g) ground cumin

½ teaspoon (1 g) ground coriander

½ teaspoon (2 g) garlic powder

½ teaspoon (1 g) onion powder

½ teaspoon (3 g) salt

½ teaspoon (1 g) pepper

Cook, then add:

8 ounces (225 g) shrimp, cooked

½ cup (120 ml) full fat sour cream

½ cup (50 g) grated Cheddar

(*1,070 calories, 31 grams net carbs*)

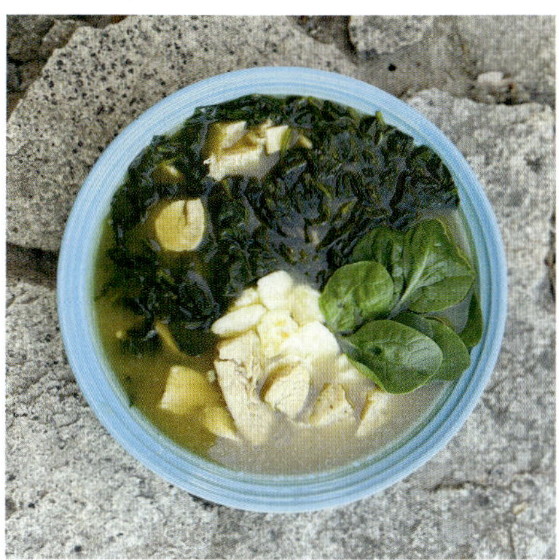

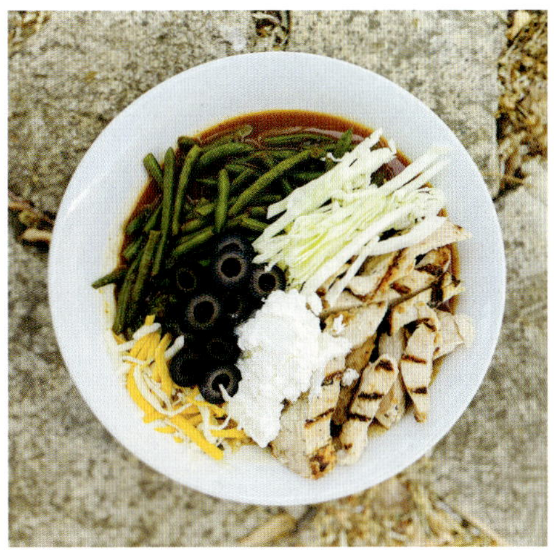

Saag Paneer–Style Soup with Chicken

8 ounces (225 g) chicken breast, cooked
12 ounces (340 g) frozen spinach
2 cups (470 ml) chicken broth
½ cup (120 ml) coconut cream
½ teaspoon (2 g) garlic powder
½ teaspoon (1 g) onion powder
½ teaspoon (3 g) salt
½ teaspoon (1 g) pepper
½ teaspoon (1 g) ginger powder
2 teaspoons (4 g) ground cumin
2 teaspoons (3 g) garam masala
½ teaspoon (2 g) turmeric
⅛ teaspoon (¼ g) cayenne
½ cup (60 g) paneer or a Mexican frying cheese
(*910 calories, 22 grams net carbs*)

Chicken Enchilada Soup

8 ounces (225 g) chicken, cooked
12 ounces (340 g) frozen green beans
3 cups (710 ml) chicken broth
1 teaspoon (3 g) chili powder
1 teaspoon (2 g) ground cumin
½ teaspoon (2 g) garlic powder
½ teaspoon (1 g) onion powder
½ teaspoon (3 g) salt
½ teaspoon (2 g) pepper
½ teaspoon (1 g) ground oregano

Cook, then add:

½ cup (50 g) grated Cheddar
½ cup (120 ml) sour cream
8 olives
(*1,025 calories, 28 grams net carbs*)

chapter seven

Pureed Soup

This is a highly formulaic and simple meal type that uses the same cooking method as the skillet and soup recipes, except that it adds one additional step—pureeing the ingredients. Experiment with the texture of these recipes. A popular variation, for instance, is to make the clam chowder but add the clams at the end so they are not pureed. It is all about finding the variety that you crave.

THE BASIC PUREED SOUP PROCESS

In each of the recipes below, gather all ingredients in the top portion of the recipe (all of those above the line "Cook, puree, then add"). Warm your skillet on medium high. Combine the main vegetable and meat ingredients in the skillet.

Make your sauce by mixing the seasonings in a bowl with the broth: stir them together well before adding to the skillet. In this step, include any extras for the sauce, such as the tomato paste or peanut powder.

Add the sauce to the skillet. Cover. Cook for 10 to 20 minutes until the vegetables are cooked. (Time will depend on your quantity and your stove.)

Place the skillet ingredients in a blender or food processor and puree.

Add the ingredients in the lower part of the recipe, stirring in items such as cream. Cheese and garnishes can be sprinkled on top or mixed in, as you desire. Adjust for salt and pepper.

Note: All the following recipes are for a single serving and should constitute your single meal or total caloric intake for the day.

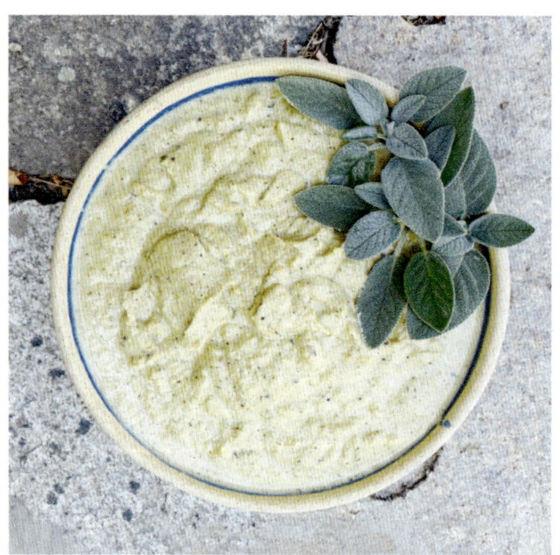

Cream of Broccoli Soup

8 ounces (225 g) chicken breast, cooked
12 ounces (340 g) frozen broccoli
2 cups (470 ml) chicken broth
½ teaspoon (2 g) garlic powder
½ teaspoon (1 g) onion powder
½ teaspoon (3 g) salt
½ teaspoon (1 g) pepper
½ teaspoon (1 g) ground basil
¼ teaspoon (½ g) paprika
⅛ teaspoon (¼ g) ground mustard
½ teaspoon (1 g) celery seed

Cook, puree, then add:

½ cup (120 ml) cream
½ cup (50 g) grated Cheddar
(*1,150 calories, 19 grams net carbs*)

Asian Spinach Soup

1 tablespoon (15 ml) cooking oil
8 ounces (225 g) chicken, cooked
12 ounces (340 g) frozen spinach
3 cups (710 ml) chicken broth
1 cup (240 ml) coconut milk
½ teaspoon (2 g) garlic powder
½ teaspoon (1 g) onion powder
½ teaspoon (3 g) salt
½ teaspoon (1 g) pepper
3 tablespoons (18 g) peanut powder

Cook, puree, then add:

2 teaspoons (10 ml) apple cider vinegar
(*1,145 calories, 15 grams net carbs*)

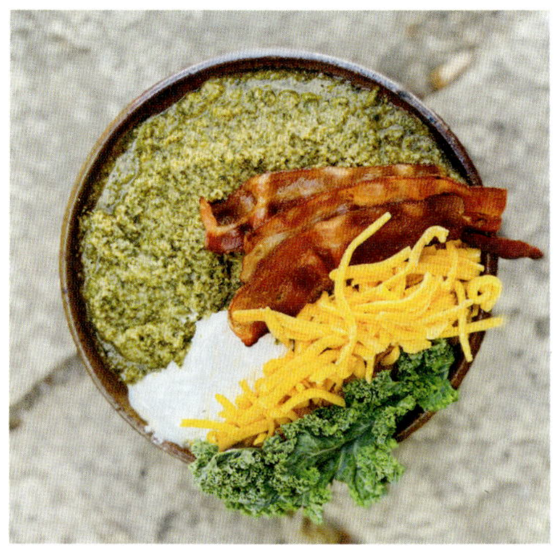

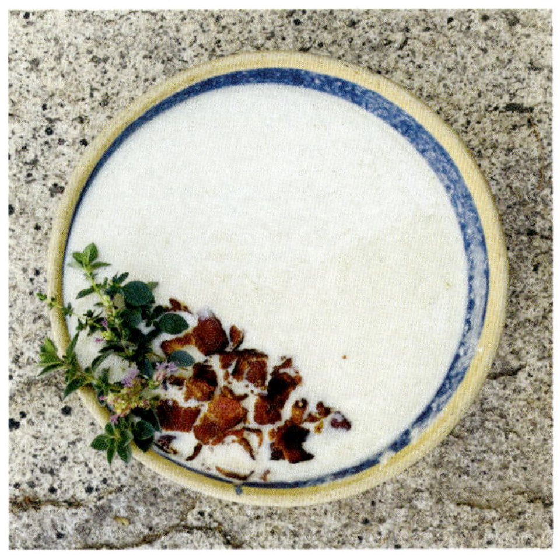

Kale and Sausage

1 tablespoon (15 ml) cooking oil
5 ounces (140 g) sausage (Italian or chorizo), cooked
8 ounces (225 g) frozen cauliflower
4 ounces (115 g) frozen kale
2 cups (470 ml) beef broth
1 tablespoon (2 g) dried parsley
½ teaspoon (2 g) garlic powder
½ teaspoon (1 g) onion powder
½ teaspoon (3 g) salt
½ teaspoon (1 g) pepper

Cook, puree, then add:

½ cup (50 g) grated Cheddar
1 tablespoon (15 ml) sour cream
4 slices bacon
(*1,040 calories, 15 grams net carbs*)

Clam Chowder

1 tablespoon (15 ml) cooking oil
6 ounce (180 g) can clams
8 ounces (225 g) frozen cauliflower
4 stalks celery, chopped
2 cups (470 ml) chicken broth
½ teaspoon (2 g) garlic powder
½ teaspoon (1 g) onion powder
½ teaspoon (3 g) salt
½ teaspoon (1 g) pepper
½ teaspoon (1 g) dried thyme

Cook, puree, then add:

½ cup (120 ml) cream
¼ cup (30 g) grated Parmesan
4 slices crisp bacon
1 teaspoon (5 ml) apple cider vinegar
(*1,050 calories, 13 grams net carbs*)

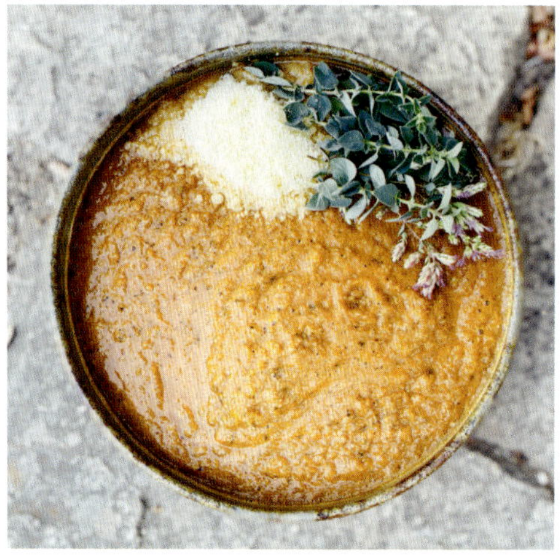

Minestrone

1 tablespoon (15 ml) cooking oil
8 ounces (225 g) sausage (Italian or chorizo), cooked
8 ounces (225 g) frozen cauliflower
4 stalks celery, chopped
2 cups (470 ml) beef broth
2 tablespoons (30 ml) tomato paste
1 teaspoon (1 g) ground basil
1 teaspoon (2 g) ground oregano
1 teaspoon (½ g) dried parsley
½ teaspoon (2 g) garlic powder
½ teaspoon (1 g) onion powder
½ teaspoon (3 g) salt
½ teaspoon (1 g) pepper

Cook, puree, then add:

¼ cup (30 g) grated Parmesan
(*1,070 calories, 18 grams net carbs*)

Chili

1 tablespoon (15 ml) cooking oil
8 ounces (225 g) ground beef, cooked
12 ounces (340 g) frozen cauliflower
2 cups (470 ml) beef broth
2 tablespoons (30 ml) tomato paste
½ teaspoon (2 g) garlic powder
½ teaspoon (1 g) onion powder
½ teaspoon (3 g) salt
½ teaspoon (1 g) pepper
½ teaspoon (1 g) ground basil
1 tablespoon (9 g) chili powder
½ teaspoon (1 g) ground cumin

Cook, puree, then add:

1 tablespoon (15 ml) sour cream
2 tablespoons (20 g) sliced olives
¼ cup (25 g) grated Cheddar
(*1,010 calories, 17 grams net carbs*)

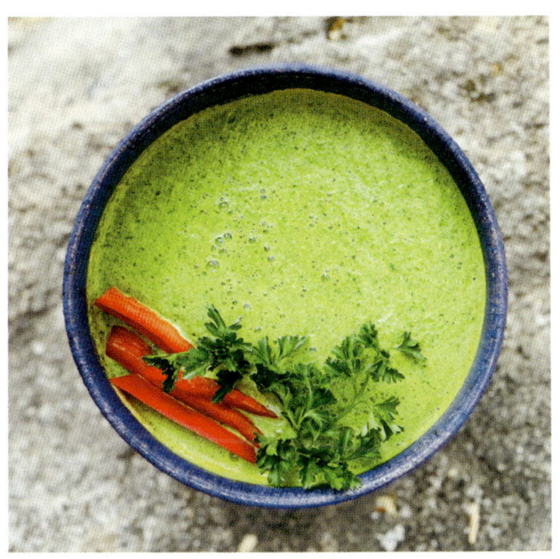

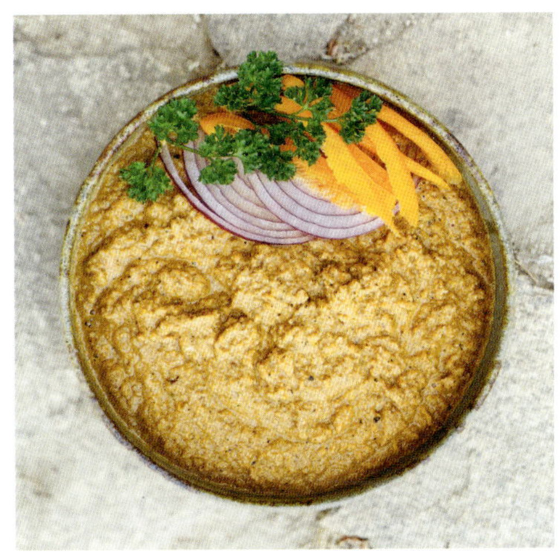

Collard Greens Curry Soup

1 tablespoon (15 ml) cooking oil
8 ounces (225 g) chicken, cooked
12 ounces (340 g) frozen collard greens
1 quart (1 liter) chicken broth
½ teaspoon (2 g) garlic powder
½ teaspoon (1 g) onion powder
½ teaspoon (3 g) salt
½ teaspoon (1 g) pepper

Cook, puree, then add:
½ cup (120 ml) cream
(*1,060 calories, 16 grams net carbs*)

Creole

2 tablespoons (30 ml) cooking oil
8 ounces (225 g) ground beef, cooked
12 ounces (340 g) frozen cauliflower
2 cups (470 ml) beef broth
1 tablespoon (15 ml) tomato paste
½ teaspoon (2 g) garlic powder
½ teaspoon (1 g) onion powder
½ teaspoon (3 g) salt
½ teaspoon (1 g) pepper
¼ teaspoon (½ g) cayenne
1 tablespoon (5 g) ground basil
1 teaspoon (5 g) horseradish powder, optional

Cook, puree, then add:
1 bell pepper, chopped
(*950 calories, 22 grams net carbs*)

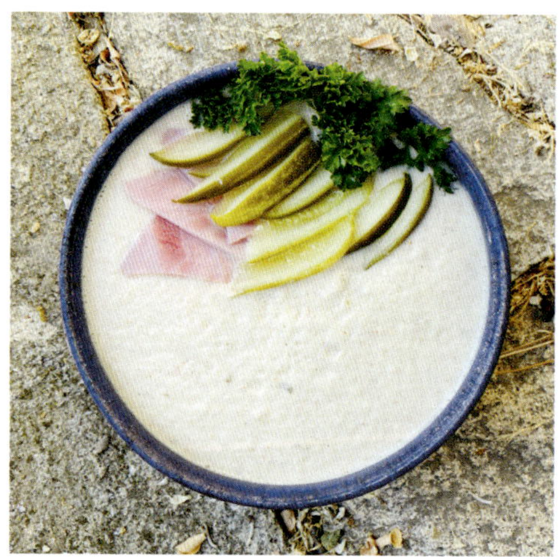

Pickle Soup

1 tablespoon (15 ml) cooking oil
8 ounces (225 g) ham, cooked
12 ounces (340 g) frozen cauliflower
2 cups (470 ml) chicken broth
½ cup (120 ml) dill pickle juice
¾ cup (130 g) pickles, chopped (about two large dills)
½ teaspoon (2 g) garlic powder
½ teaspoon (1 g) onion powder
½ teaspoon (3 g) salt
½ teaspoon (1 g) pepper
⅛ teaspoon (¼ g) cayenne

Cook, puree, then add:

½ cup (120 ml) cream or sour cream
(*1,050 calories, 20 grams net carbs*)

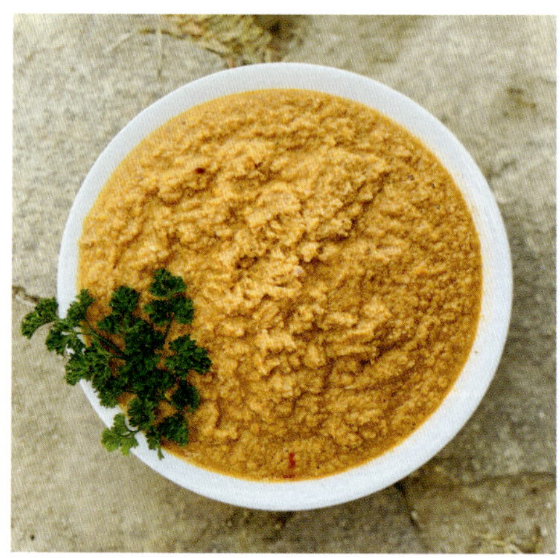

Goulash

1 tablespoon (15 ml) cooking oil
8 ounces (225 g) ground beef, cooked
12 ounces (340 g) frozen cauliflower
2 cups (470 ml) chicken broth
1 tablespoon (15 ml) tomato paste
½ teaspoon (2 g) garlic powder
½ teaspoon (1 g) onion powder
½ teaspoon (3 g) salt
½ teaspoon (1 g) pepper
1 teaspoon (2 g) paprika
½ teaspoon (1 g) caraway seed

Cook, puree, then add:

6 slices of bacon, chopped
(*1,090 calories, 13 grams net carbs*)

chapter eight

Konjac Noodles

Konjac is a yam that, by some process, gets turned into a noodle-like food. Konjac is also known as glucomannan and comes in the form of a powder that you may use as a thickener. This is a very high-fiber item that has zero calories. The noodle definitely has haters (and you may be one of them). The noodles look just like rice noodles when cooked, and so your brain will expect rice noodles. However, the texture is more in the rubber-band-texture category, and that will be a big turnoff for many people. The noodles also tend to have a fishy flavor, but you can take care of that problem in your preparation.

THE BASIC KONJAC PROCESS

For these dishes, you need to prepare the noodles in advance. Drain them from their package and rinse them well under running water in a colander or strainer. Next, dry-fry them in a hot skillet for about 5 minutes. You are basically drying some of the fishy moisture out of them. After dry-frying, the noodles will absorb some of the flavor of the sauce, but they will still have a bit of a chewy texture.

I typically make the sauce while the noodles are dry-frying and add it to the noodles. I add the protein at this point, and I might add an extra vegetable, like green beans. If your protein is frozen, turn the heat down and put a lid on the skillet to allow the protein to simmer until it has defrosted.

Note: All the following recipes are for a single serving and should constitute your single meal or total caloric intake for the day.

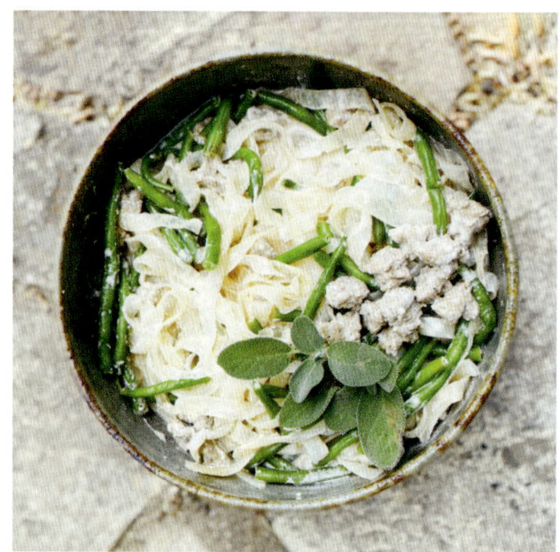

Sausage Gravy over Noodles

8 ounces (225 g) sausage, cooked
4 ounces (115 g) frozen green beans, optional
14 ounces (400 g) konjac noodles (2 packages)
½ cup (120 ml) chicken broth
½ teaspoon (2 g) garlic powder
½ teaspoon (1 g) onion powder
½ teaspoon (3 g) salt
½ teaspoon (1 g) pepper

Cook, then add:
½ cup (120 ml) cream
(*1,150 calories, 11 grams net carbs*)

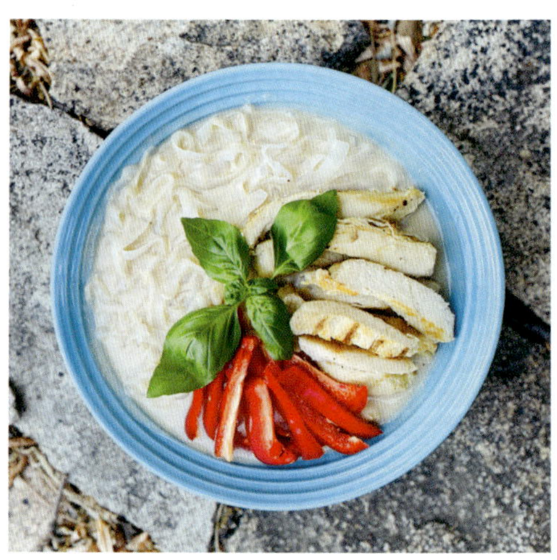

Chicken Alfredo over Noodles

8 ounces (225 g) chicken, cooked
14 ounces (400 g) konjac noodles (2 packages)
½ cup (120 ml) broth
½ teaspoon (2 g) garlic powder
½ teaspoon (1 g) onion powder
½ teaspoon (3 g) salt
½ teaspoon (1 g) pepper

Cook, then add:
½ cup (120 ml) cream
¼ cup (30 g) grated Parmesan
(*900 calories, 8 grams net carbs*)

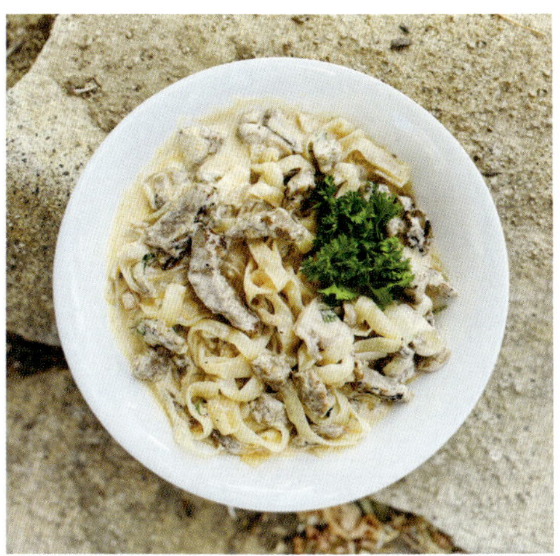

Beef Stroganoff

8 ounces (225 g) beef strips (or ground beef), cooked
4 ounces (115 g) canned mushrooms, drained
14 ounces (400 g) konjac noodles (2 packages)
½ cup (120 ml) beef broth
1 tablespoon (2 g) dried parsley
½ teaspoon (2 g) garlic powder
½ teaspoon (1 g) onion powder
½ teaspoon (3 g) salt
½ teaspoon (1 g) pepper
½ teaspoon (1 g) paprika

Cook, then add:

½ cup (120 ml) sour cream
1 tablespoon (15 ml) vinegar
(*850 calories, 9 grams net carbs*)

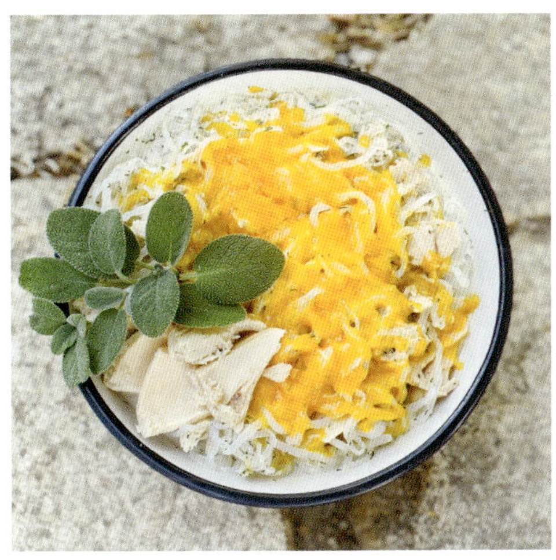

Tuna Noodle

8 ounces (225 g) canned tuna, drained
14 ounces (400 g) konjac noodles (2 packages)
¼ cup (60 ml) chicken broth
½ teaspoon (2 g) garlic powder
½ teaspoon (1 g) onion powder
½ teaspoon (3 g) salt
½ teaspoon (1 g) pepper
1 tablespoon (3 g) dried dill

Cook, then add:

½ cup (50 g) grated Cheddar
1 medium avocado, sliced
(*975 calories, 6 grams net carbs*)

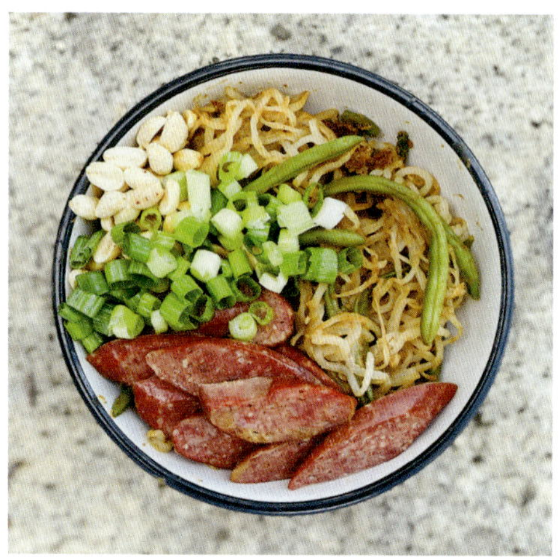

Peanut Pork

8 ounces (225 g) sausage, cooked
14 ounces (400 g) konjac noodles (2 packages)
¼ cup (60 ml) chicken broth
2 tablespoons (30 ml) soy sauce/tamari
¼ teaspoon (1 ml) sesame oil
4 tablespoons (24 g) peanut powder
½ teaspoon (2 g) garlic powder
½ teaspoon (1 g) onion powder
½ teaspoon (1 g) pepper

Cook, then add:

Green onions, sliced, for garnish, optional
Peanuts for garnish, optional
(*900 calories, 8 grams net carbs*)

chapter nine

Recipe Variations

THE VEGETARIAN VARIATION

The RBS recipes are extremely easy to adapt to a vegetarian or completely plant-based way of eating. In many cases, you simply need to swap the protein with a lower-carbohydrate plant-based option. Many of the Veggie Bear communities lean on tofu and soy-based products of various kinds. In those cases, adapt the cooking method slightly depending on best practices for that particular protein item. There are many that will simply need to be heated in the skillet. Tofu would benefit from being fried and then immersed in the sauce of the dish so that it can take on its flavor.

Some community members are eating beans and bean products of various kinds as the protein. These have higher levels of carbohydrates, but they may be a completely adequate solution to help you reach your goal. That is for you to experiment with.

If you are implementing a one-meal model, and especially if you are plant based, you may have to work at hitting a calorie level above 800. Whereas most of us need to be concerned about adding too much, you might look for avocados and nuts to boost the calories and help you feel more satisfied. People who eat dairy will have no problem here; cheese or sour cream gets you there pretty quickly.

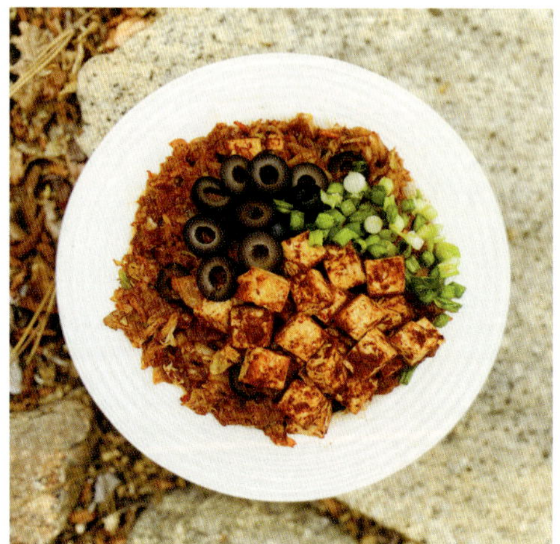

Veggie Taco Bowl

2 tablespoons (30 ml) cooking oil

8 ounces (225 g) tofu, cubed, fried, and added to sauce

½ head cabbage, chopped

¼ cup (60 ml) vegetable broth

½ teaspoon (2 g) garlic powder

½ teaspoon (1 g) onion powder

½ teaspoon (3 g) salt

½ teaspoon (1 g) pepper

1 teaspoon (3 g) chili powder

1 teaspoon (2 g) ground cumin

1/8 teaspoon (¼ g) cayenne

½ teaspoon (1 g) ground oregano

Cook, then add:

½ cup (50 g) grated Cheddar

(900 calories, 25 grams net carbs)

As written, this is the regular taco bowl from the sauté recipe collection, except that it has tofu and a bit more cooking oil. Add a medium avocado for about an additional 300 calories and about 4 grams of carbohydrates.

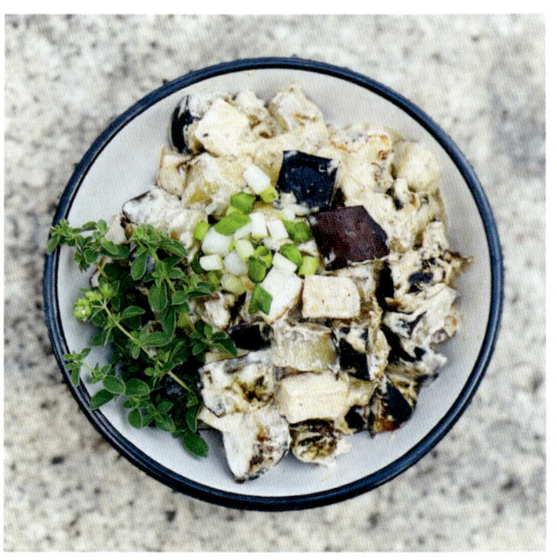

Eggplant and Gravy

1 tablespoon (15 ml) cooking oil

8 ounces (225 g) tofu, cubed, fried, and added to sauce

12 ounces (340 g) frozen eggplant

½ cup (120 ml) vegetable broth

½ cup (120 ml) coconut cream

½ teaspoon (2 g) garlic powder

½ teaspoon (1 g) onion powder

½ teaspoon (3 g) salt

½ teaspoon (1 g) pepper

Cook, then add:

1 medium avocado, sliced

(1,170 calories, 25 grams net carbs)

THE LOWER-CALORIE VARIATION

Particularly if you are eating two meals a day, you will want to reduce the calories in each. Many of the recipes in this book can easily have calories shaved off, particularly if there is cream or cheese in the recipe. A fattier meat can be replaced with something leaner like shrimp or chicken breasts. Simply reduce or cut out these more calorie-dense ingredients, leaving a dish much like the extra-lean Cajun Shrimp or Chicken Teriyaki dishes.

You will also find some lower-calorie options throughout this book, but you can craft any low-calorie dish with some of these basic changes.

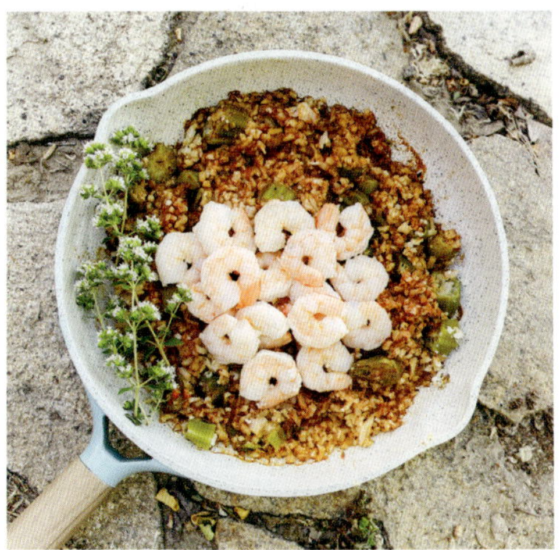

Cajun Shrimp over Cauliflower Rice

1 tablespoon (15 ml) cooking oil
10 ounces (300 g) frozen cauliflower rice
4 ounces (115 g) frozen okra or green beans
½ cup (120 ml) chicken broth
1 tablespoon (15 ml) tomato paste
½ teaspoon (2 g) garlic powder
½ teaspoon (1 g) onion powder
½ teaspoon (3 g) salt
½ teaspoon (1 g) pepper
¼ teaspoon (1 g) chili powder
½ teaspoon (1 g) ground oregano
¼ teaspoon (1 g) ground thyme
1 teaspoon (2 g) paprika

Cook, then add:

8 ounces (225 g) shrimp, cooked
(510 calories, 18 grams net carbs)

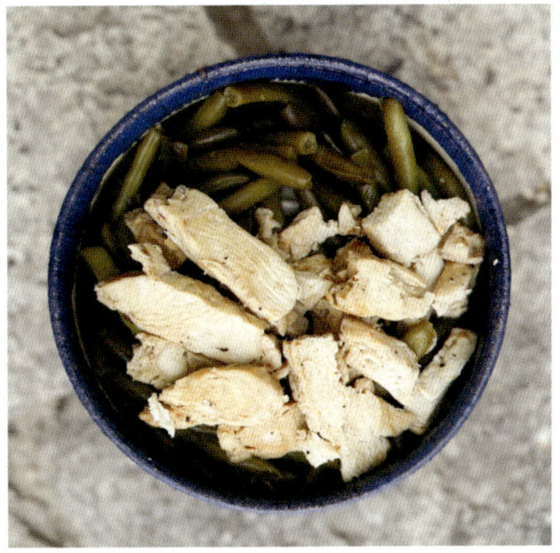

Chicken Teriyaki Green Beans

1 tablespoon (15 ml) cooking oil
8 ounces (225 g) chicken breast, cooked
12 ounces (340 g) frozen green beans
½ cup (120 ml) chicken broth
2 tablespoons (30 ml) soy sauce/tamari
½ tablespoon (7 ml) apple cider vinegar
½ teaspoon (2 g) garlic powder
½ teaspoon (1 g) onion powder
½ teaspoon (1 g) pepper
½ teaspoon (1 g) ginger powder
¼ teaspoon (1 g) chili pepper
(650 calories, 20 grams net carbs)

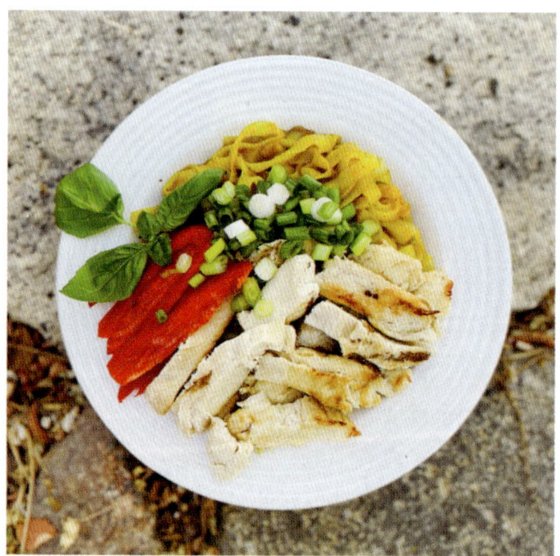

Curry Chicken Noodle

8 ounces (225 g) chicken, cooked
14 ounces (400 g) konjac noodles (2 packages)
1 cup (240 ml) chicken broth
½ teaspoon (2 g) garlic powder
½ teaspoon (1 g) ginger powder
½ teaspoon (3 g) salt
½ teaspoon (1 g) pepper
½ teaspoon (1 g) ground coriander
½ teaspoon (1 g) ground cumin
¼ teaspoon (1 g) turmeric
⅛ teaspoon (¼ g) cayenne
⅛ teaspoon (½ g) annatto, optional
1 teaspoon (5 g) glucomannan powder, optional
Sweetener to taste, optional

Cook, then add:

Green onions, sliced, optional
(*400 calories, 3 grams net carbs*)

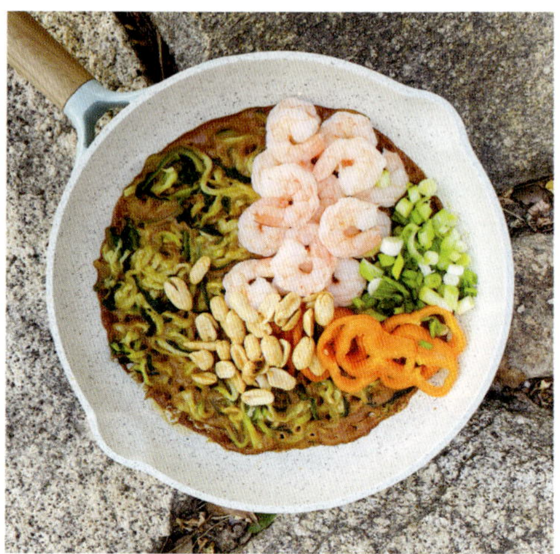

Peanut Shrimp over Zoodles

1 tablespoon (15 ml) cooking oil
12 ounces (340 g) frozen zoodles
¼ cup (60 ml) chicken broth
2 tablespoons (30 ml) soy sauce/tamari
1 teaspoon (5 ml) sesame oil
4 tablespoons (24 g) peanut powder
½ teaspoon (2 g) garlic powder
½ teaspoon (1 g) onion powder
½ teaspoon (1 g) pepper

Cook, then add:

8 ounces (225 g) shrimp, cooked
Green onions and bell pepper, chopped for garnish, optional
(*540 calories, 17 grams net carbs*)

THE "DON'T COMPLETELY OVERCOOK IT" VARIATION (SHRIMP)

Sometimes you will have situations where you may overcook or dry out your protein if you add it to the pan in the beginning. Shrimp is a key example. Most of us purchase it already cooked, and it can very quickly get overcooked and chewy if it is cooked along with the other ingredients. In cases like this, just add it in the last few minutes, usually with a lid on the pan to contain the heat. Turn off the heat after a few minutes and let it sit a few more if you want to ensure that the protein is warm.

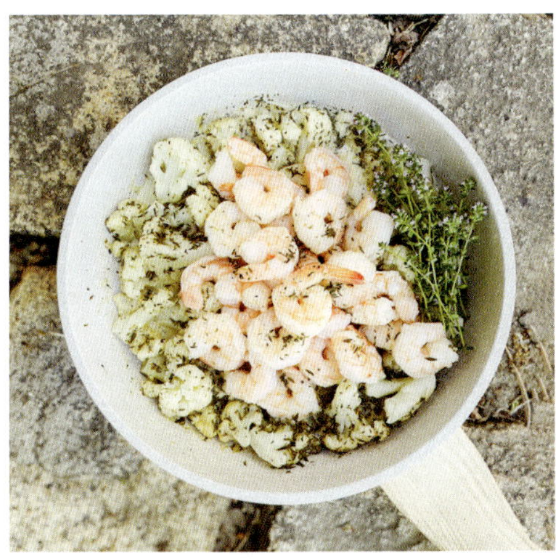

Creamy Herb Shrimp over Cauliflower

1 tablespoon (15 ml) cooking oil
12 ounces (340 g) frozen cauliflower
½ cup (120 ml) chicken broth
½ teaspoon (2 g) garlic powder
½ teaspoon (1 g) onion powder
½ teaspoon (3 g) salt
½ teaspoon (1 g) pepper
2 tablespoons (12 g) ground oregano or basil

Cook, then add:

8 ounces (225 g) shrimp, cooked
½ cup (120 g) ricotta
½ cup (60 g) grated Parmesan
Pine nuts for garnish, optional
(900 calories, 21 grams net carbs)

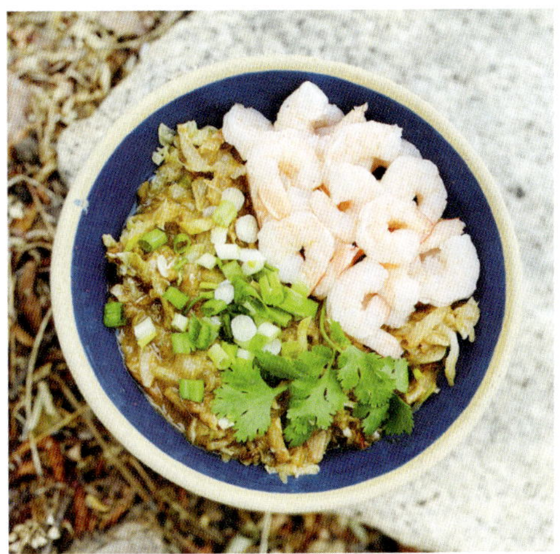

Peanut Shrimp Skillet

2 tablespoons (30 ml) cooking oil
½ head cabbage, chopped
¼ cup (60 ml) chicken broth
2 tablespoons (30 ml) soy sauce/tamari
1 tablespoon (15 ml) sesame oil
4 tablespoons (24 g) peanut powder
½ teaspoon (2 g) garlic powder
½ teaspoon (1 g) onion powder
½ teaspoon (1 g) pepper
Sweetener to taste, optional

Cook, then add:

8 ounces (225 g) shrimp, cooked
(870 calories, 23 grams net carbs)

THE FROZEN/RAW PROTEIN VARIATION (FISH)

You can definitely start with a raw protein item and cook it in the skillet itself. The obvious application is frozen raw fish. These days, frozen fish often comes raw in vacuum-sealed plastic bags for easy single-serving uses. The best approach to cooking frozen fish in these dishes is to place the fish on the bottom of the skillet, pile the vegetables on top, and then pour over the sauce. The sauce will help keep the fish from drying out. If the fish has skin (as salmon often does), place it skin side up to keep the moisture in the fish. Allow about 20 minutes to cook and check the fish for doneness. It should flake away with a fork when it is cooked. Fish is easy to overcook, but the moisture in these dishes helps keep it from drying out.

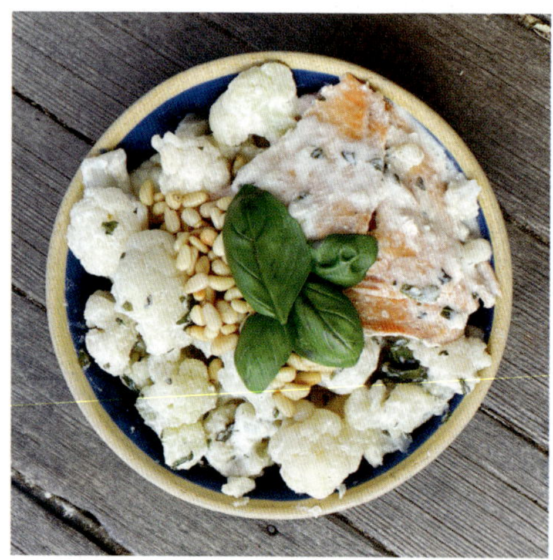

Basil Salmon over Cauliflower

1 tablespoon (15 ml) cooking oil
8 ounces (225 g) frozen raw salmon
12 ounces (340 g) frozen cauliflower
½ cup (120 ml) chicken broth
½ teaspoon (2 g) garlic powder
½ teaspoon (1 g) onion powder
½ teaspoon (3 g) salt
½ teaspoon (1 g) pepper
2 tablespoons (9 g) ground basil

Cook, then add:

½ cup (120 g) ricotta
½ cup (60 g) grated Parmesan
Pine nuts for garnish, optional
(*1,090 calories, 16 grams net carbs*)

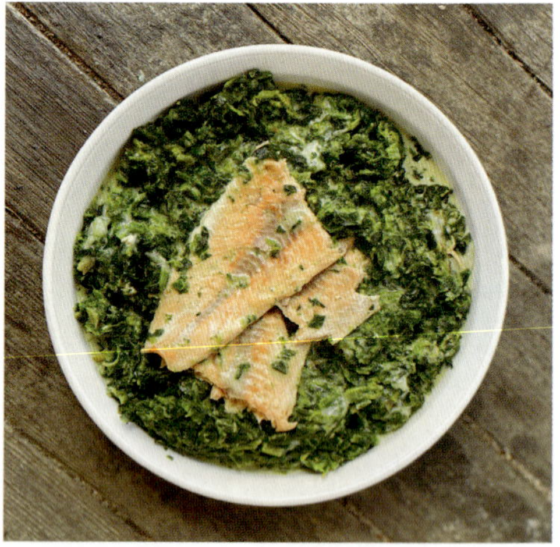

Creamy Salmon with Spinach

1 tablespoon (15 ml) cooking oil
8 ounces (225 g) frozen raw salmon fillet
12 ounces (340 g) frozen spinach
½ cup (120 ml) chicken broth
½ teaspoon (2 g) garlic powder
½ teaspoon (1 g) onion powder
½ teaspoon (3 g) salt
½ teaspoon (1 g) pepper

Cook, then add:

½ cup (120 ml) cream
(*1,067 calories, 10 grams net carbs*)

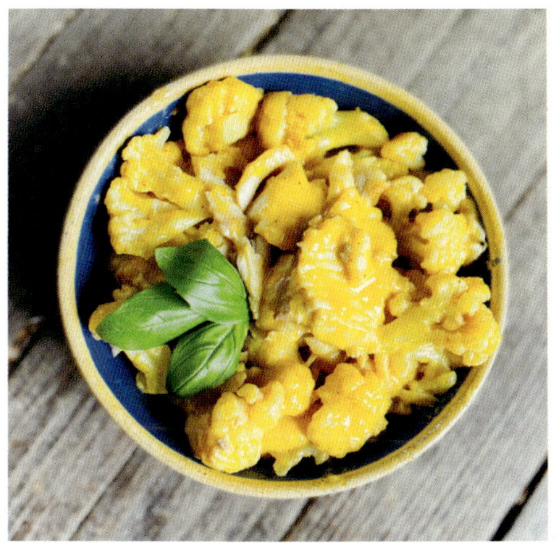

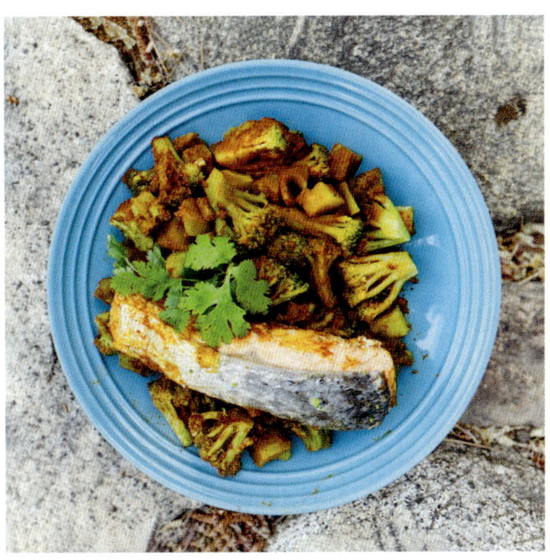

Panang Fish

1 tablespoon (15 ml) cooking oil
8 ounces (225 g) frozen raw cod (or other fish)
12 ounces (340 g) frozen cauliflower
½ cup (120 ml) coconut cream
½ teaspoon (2 g) garlic powder
½ teaspoon (1 g) onion powder
½ teaspoon (3 g) salt
½ teaspoon (1 g) pepper
½ teaspoon (1 g) ground coriander
½ teaspoon (1 g) ground cumin
¼ teaspoon (1 g) turmeric
⅛ teaspoon (¼ g) cayenne
⅛ teaspoon (½ g) annatto (optional)
Sweetener to taste, optional
(*920 calories, 25 grams net carbs*)

Salmon Masala

1 tablespoon (15 ml) cooking oil
8 ounces (225 g) frozen raw salmon
12 ounces (340 g) frozen broccoli
½ cup (120 ml) chicken or fish broth
2 tablespoons (30 ml) tomato paste
½ teaspoon (2 g) garlic powder
½ teaspoon (1 g) onion powder
½ teaspoon (3 g) salt
½ teaspoon (1 g) pepper
1 teaspoon (2 g) ginger powder
1 teaspoon (2 g) garam masala
1 teaspoon (2 g) ground coriander
1 teaspoon (2 g) ground cumin
⅛ teaspoon (¼ g) cayenne

Cook, then add:
½ cup (120 ml) sour cream
(*1,020 calories, 28 grams net carbs*)

THE "USE CANNED SAUCE" VARIATION

It's almost against my religion to post these recipes, but people often ask if they can use canned sauces and dressings. You can use anything you wish. With canned sauces, we often end up with a few more grams of carbohydrates than we would with homemade, but that is far better than the drive-through.

The pesto concept below can be an excellent option for getting extra basil flavor in your dishes in a very convenient way. It is also easy to make pesto yourself, but there really are some good pesto options on the market. Check the carbs on the packaging.

Enchilada sauce is easily found in any grocery store and brings a quick Mexican flavor to your dishes. It is also extremely easy to make yourself, and you will find a homemade enchilada version here in this book. If you keep those spices in your cupboard, you will always be about a minute away from the homemade version.

Jarred Alfredo sauce is available in any grocery store and a quick convenient option. However, you will laugh when you find the homemade version in this book. Keep cream and Parmesan on hand to make this sauce easily at home. Check the carbs on the product.

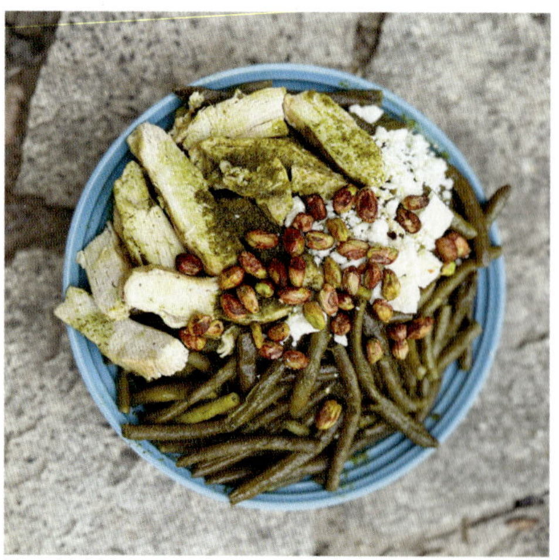

Pesto Chicken

8 ounces (225 g) chicken breast, cooked
12 ounces (340 g) frozen green beans
½ cup (120 ml) chicken broth
¼ cup (60 ml) pesto
½ teaspoon (2 g) garlic powder
½ teaspoon (1 g) onion powder
½ teaspoon (3 g) salt
½ teaspoon (1 g) pepper

Cook, then add:

4 ounces (115 g) goat cheese
Nuts, optional
(1,115 calories, 17 grams net carbs)

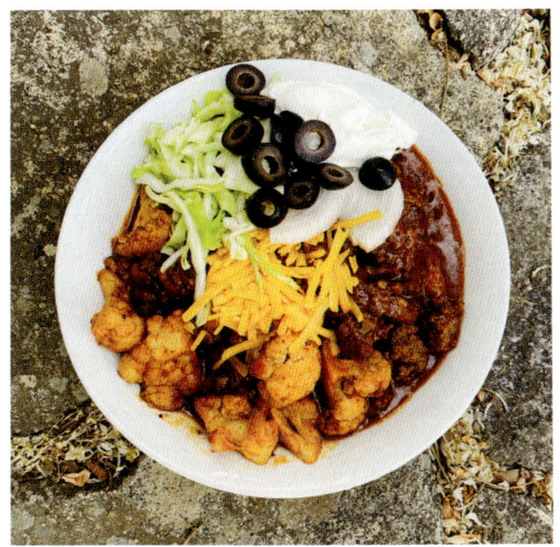

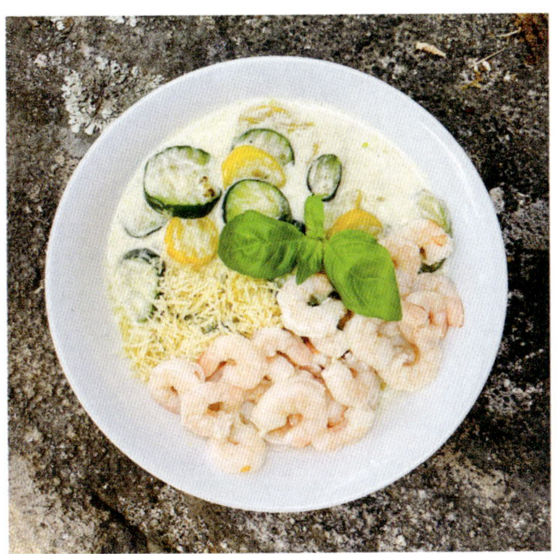

Enchilada Skillet

6 ounces (170 g) ground beef, cooked
12 ounces (340 g) frozen cauliflower
½ cup (120 ml) beef broth
5 ounces (150 ml) canned enchilada sauce
½ teaspoon (1 g) onion powder
½ teaspoon (2 g) garlic powder
½ teaspoon (3 g) salt
½ teaspoon (1 g) pepper

Cook, then add:

½ cup (120 ml) full-fat sour cream
½ cup (50 g) grated Cheddar
(*1,220 calories, 18 grams net carbs*)

Shrimp Alfredo over Summer Squash

12 ounces (340 g) frozen summer squash
½ cup (120 ml) chicken broth
½ teaspoon (3 g) salt
½ teaspoon (1 g) pepper
½ cup (120 ml) jarred Alfredo sauce
½ teaspoon (3 g) glucomannan

Cook, then add:

8 ounces (225 g) shrimp, cooked
(*850 calories, 24 grams net carbs*)

chapter ten

Your Six-Week Plan

Based on the popularity of the Six-Week Plan in the first RBS book, I offer you a Six-Week Ridiculously Big Skillet Plan. I will admit right here that I would basically never follow any sort of specific Six-Week Plan for cooking. I would jump into this list and cherry-pick it. You may choose to do so as well.

In making this plan, I started with basic recipes that require few seasonings. I also started with just a couple of protein items and then increased the variety over the six weeks. I figure that allows you some time to build up your stash of freezer items if you choose. You may not need to buy a particular protein item again for a few weeks if you cooked a big batch of it in an earlier week. That is essentially what I do all the time, but not knowing what opportunities or sales might arise, I allow myself a whole lot of flexibility. That flexibility is why I personally would cherry-pick this list.

However, the Six-Week Plan is also a time to taste a wide variety of recipes, so there is definitely value in getting through many of these recipes.

Unlike the first RBS book, I am adding pantry items here week by week to reduce your cost each time you shop.

MY HOPE WITH THIS SIX-WEEK PLAN

My hope and purpose in this chapter is to expose you to an array of flavors and combinations so that, hopefully, a few will rise to the top as your "easy favorites" I discussed earlier. I try to do this in a way that is budget-friendly as you build your pantry, should this book find your pantry bare.

In the process of whipping up these recipes every single day, you will also develop a keen sense of the parts and components themselves—the framework aspect of the meals. Get a good instinct for the bulk of the vegetables and the amount of additional fat and protein, and you really will get to a point of tossing together a flavorful meal with very little thought, one that will help you reach your long-term goals.

As for the sequence in these six weeks of meals, there is nothing particularly special in the order here, except that I have tried to keep things simpler at first as you build out your pantry and freezer items. There are more prepared meats on the front end of the plan as you build—for instance, ham and sausage. They are there for convenience. Just regular pork cuts may be a healthier choice, but getting and staying on track is the most critical aspect in all of this. Over time, you can fill your freezer with all sorts of alternatives.

WEEK 1

This is an exciting week because you do begin to build out a nice little stash of items in your pantry and freezer. This week, if you're into batch cooking, I encourage you to cook chicken breasts and add them to your stash. I tend to freeze them in strips for these recipes, because most recipes call for strips. However, you can certainly use them whole or even shredded.

I have added both sausage and ham to the list this week primarily to give you a jump on the protein. These are already cooked and, as a result, more in the convenience category. The sausage this week can be any sort of sausage you like that pairs with the sweet and salty flavors of teriyaki (which, frankly, is most sausage). If you stumble upon a large ham at a good price, you can slice it and freeze it in usable quantities.

WEEK 1 MEALS

Ham and Cheese Soup (69)
Chicken Teriyaki (53)
Chicken Alfredo (64)
Chicken Mushroom Casserole (52)
Sausage Cauliflower Teriyaki (55)
Pickle Soup (78)
Pork Faux Rice (62)

WEEK 1 SHOPPING LIST

Pantry Items

Salt
Pepper
Garlic powder
Ginger powder
Onion powder
Oregano
Paprika
Cooking oil
Sesame oil
Soy sauce
Apple cider vinegar
Sweetener

Protein

16 ounces (450 g) ham
24 ounces (680 g) chicken breast
12 ounces (340 g) sausage

Vegetables

1 head cabbage
24 ounces (680 g) broccoli
16 ounces (450 g) frozen green beans
24 ounces (680 g) frozen cauliflower
10 ounces (280 g) frozen cauliflower rice

Other

2 quarts (2 liters) chicken broth
1½ cups (360 ml) cream
¼ cup (60 g) grated Parmesan
1 cup (100 g) grated Cheddar
4 ounces (115 g) canned mushrooms, drained
½ cup (60 g) peanuts
Dill pickles
Green onions
2 eggs

WEEK 2

I keep a good bit of prepared beef in my own freezer, in freezer bags in quantities that I tend to use in one meal. If you are inclined to do the same, this is the week for you. This week, grab some bulk beef and cook

WEEK 2 MEALS

Beef Stroganoff (55)
Korean Beef (56)
Eggroll in a Bowl (60)
Beef Teriyaki (56)
Peanut Shrimp Skillet (87)
Asian Spinach Soup (74)
Sausage and Mushroom Gravy (54)

WEEK 2 SHOPPING LIST

Pantry items

Peanut powder

Protein

24 ounces (680 g) beef strips (or ground beef)
16 ounces (450 g) ground sausage
8 ounces (225 g) shrimp
8 ounces (225 g) chicken

Vegetables

36 ounces (1,020 g) frozen cauliflower
1 head cabbage
12 ounces (340 g) frozen broccoli
12 ounces (340 g) frozen spinach
Green onions and cucumber, optional

Other

4 ounces (115 g) canned mushrooms
1½ cup (360 ml) beef broth
1 quart (1 liter) chicken broth
½ cup (120 ml) sour cream
½ cup (120 ml) cream
1 cup (240 ml) coconut milk
14 ounces (400 g) konjac noodles (2 packages)

some to eat and some to store. Each of the beef-centered meals for the week could include either beef strips or ground beef, so choose your favorite or what's on sale and go with it.

WEEK 3

My dream freezer would have salmon in it all the time, some cooked and some frozen raw. This week you can stock your freezer with cooked salmon, but you can buy it raw and store it frozen, using the cooking techniques for frozen raw protein in the skillet section of this book. You will also buy a selection of spices used in Mexican and Indian cuisine to start bringing a bit more flavor variety to your dishes.

WEEK 3 MEALS

Saag Paneer–Style Soup with Chicken (71)
Peanut Shrimp over Zoodles (86)
Chicken Enchilada Soup (71)
Cheeseburger in a Bowl (58)
Broccoli Beef Stir-Fry (60)
Basil Salmon over Cauliflower (88)
Salmon Masala (89)

WEEK 3 SHOPPING LIST

Pantry items

Basil
Cayenne
Chili powder
Coriander
Cumin
Garam masala
Oregano
Turmeric
Yellow mustard (deli mustard)

Protein

16 ounces (450 g) chicken breast
8 ounces (225 g) cooked shrimp
16 ounces (450 g) beef
16 ounces (450 g) frozen salmon
2 slices of bacon

Vegetables

12 ounces (340 g) frozen spinach
12 ounces (340 g) frozen zoodles
12 ounces (340 g) frozen green beans
24 ounces (680 g) frozen cauliflower
24 ounces (680 g) frozen broccoli
Green onions and bell pepper for garnish, optional
1 pickle spear
1 white onion

Other

7 cups (1.7 liters) chicken broth
¾ cup (180 ml) beef broth
½ cup (120 ml) coconut cream
2 tablespoons (30 ml) tomato paste
½ cup (60 g) paneer or a Mexican frying cheese
¾ cup (75 g) grated Cheddar
½ cup (120 ml) sour cream
½ cup (120 g) ricotta
½ cup (60 g) grated Parmesan
2 tablespoons (30 ml) mayonnaise
2 tablespoons (30 ml) Greek yogurt
½ teaspoon (2 ml) yellow/deli mustard
8 olives, optional
Pine nuts for garnish, optional

WEEK 4

This week you may grab some more beef to use as steak strips in these dishes. You'll have some shrimp and pork as well. This may be the time to purchase both beef and pork in bulk to add to your freezer stash. You can often find some pretty decent sales on beef and pork—an opportunity to stash a whole tower of meat-filled baggies in your freezer.

WEEK 4 MEALS

Tuna Noodle (81)
Salsa Verde Shrimp (70)
Chicken Fajita Stir-Fry (67)
Philly Cheesesteak in a Bowl (66)
Chili (76)
Minestrone (76)
Panang Chicken (52)

WEEK 4 SHOPPING LIST

Pantry items

Annatto, optional for color
Glucomannan powder, optional for thickening
Parsley, dried

Protein

16 ounces (450 g) chicken breast
8 ounces (225 g) cooked shrimp
8 ounces (225 g) steak strips
8 ounces (225 g) ground beef
8 ounces (225 g) sausage (Italian or chorizo)
8 ounces (225 g) canned tuna

Vegetables

44 ounces (1250 g) frozen cauliflower
12 ounces (340 g) cabbage
12 ounces (340 g) frozen broccoli
4 stalks celery
1 white onion, optional
1 bell pepper, optional
Green onions, optional

Other

1 quart (1 liter) chicken broth
1 quart (1 liter) beef broth
14 ounces (400 g) konjac noodles (2 packages)
¾ cup (180 ml) salsa verde
½ cup (120 ml) full-fat sour cream
2¼ cup (225 g) grated Cheddar
4 slices provolone
¼ cup (30 g) grated Parmesan
4 tablespoons (60 ml) tomato paste
1 cup (240 ml) coconut cream
½ cup (60 g) guacamole
2 tablespoons (15 g) sliced olives, optional

WEEK 5

This is a fun week with some great dishes, any number of which could end up as your favorite. The Salsa Verde Chicken is a favorite in the community. The Clam Chowder is a family favorite here, though increasingly my family tells me that I should not puree the clams themselves; you may find that as well. The flavor is great either way in my opinion.

WEEK 5 MEALS

- Clam Chowder (75)
- Beef Teriyaki (56)
- Panang Fish (89)
- Salsa Verde Chicken (58)
- Creamy Salmon with Capers (70)
- Kale and Sausage (75)
- Cream of Broccoli Soup (74)

WEEK 5 SHOPPING LIST

Pantry Items

- Celery seed
- Dijon mustard
- Thyme

Protein

- 6 ounces (180 g) canned clams
- 8 ounces (225 g) beef
- 8 ounces (225 g) frozen salmon
- 8 ounces (225 g) frozen cod or other fish
- 16 ounces (450 g) chicken breast
- 5 ounces (140 g) sausage (Italian or chorizo)
- 8 slices bacon

Vegetables

- 28 ounces (800 g) frozen cauliflower
- 4 stalks celery
- 36 ounces (1020 g) frozen broccoli
- 12 ounces (340 g) frozen okra
- 4 ounces (115 g) frozen kale

Other

- 7½ cups (1.8 liters) chicken broth
- 2½ cups (600 ml) beef broth
- ½ cup (120 ml) coconut cream
- ¾ cup (180 ml) salsa verde
- ½ cup (120 ml) sour cream
- 1½ cups (360 ml) cream
- 1¼ cups (125 g) grated Cheddar
- ¼ cup (30 g) grated Parmesan
- 2 tablespoons (15 g) capers

WEEK 6

Here in Week 6, you will make a few dishes you may not have tried before and you may choose to grill some vegetables with the Taco in a Bowl. The Reuben includes mixing up a side dressing, making it possibly the most difficult of all of these recipes, which is a bit amusing because the dressing takes just a few minutes to whip up.

WEEK 6 MEALS

- Goulash (78)
- Creole (77)
- Pizza in a Bowl (62)
- Taco in a Bowl (63)
- Sausage Gravy over Noodles (80)
- Jambalaya (65)
- Reuben in a Bowl (64)

WEEK 6 SHOPPING LIST

Pantry

- Horseradish
- Mayonnaise
- Caraway seed

Protein

- 24 ounces (680 g) ground beef
- 3 ounces (90 g) pepperoni
- 17 ounces (480 g) Italian sausage
- 8 ounces (225 g) corned beef
- 4 ounces (115 g) shrimp
- 4 slices bacon, optional

Vegetables

- 36 ounces (1020 g) frozen cauliflower
- 1 head cabbage
- 4 ounces (115 g) frozen green beans, optional
- 12 ounces (340 g) frozen broccoli
- 1 bell pepper, optional
- 1 white onion
- Small avocado

Other

- 3 cups (710 ml) chicken broth
- 3 cups (710 ml) beef broth
- 6 tablespoons (90 ml) tomato paste
- 14 ounces (400 g) konjac noodles (2 packages)
- ½ cup (50 g) grated mozzarella cheese
- ½ cup (50 g) grated Cheddar
- 2 slices Swiss cheese
- ½ cup (120 ml) cream
- 2 tablespoons (30 ml) mayonnaise
- 2 tablespoons (30 ml) Greek yogurt
- 1 tablespoon (15 ml) ketchup (no sugar added)

chapter eleven

Applications and Adaptations

Everything we do at Eat Like a Bear! is here for you to adapt to meet your needs, including the framework of the RBS recipes. You do not even have to make one of these recipes to get value out of why they are working. You could take some of the concepts and wrap them around some other food approach that will help you meet your long-term goals and live your best life. The adaptations are potentially endless. In this chapter I highlight just a few common adaptations, largely to make the point that, individually, our main focus needs to be finding something that will help us balance both the need for ongoing nutrition with our desire to get out in the world and be active.

VEGETARIAN AND VEGAN

The recipes at Eat Like a Bear! are neither vegetarian nor vegan, chiefly because the recipes are based on the way I ate to lose 140 pounds (63 kilograms), and I am neither vegetarian nor vegan. Are these recipes adaptable to plant-based eating? Absolutely. In fact, I wait patiently for more success cases to emerge from our Veggie Bears group. Perhaps you are the next.

In fact, I expect that vegetarians are naturals in being Eat Like a Bear! superstars, because many already care about their health and well-being. Those are not necessary starting points, but they are a great starting point nonetheless. Vegetarians tend to have more knowledge of food and food components, so being mindful of carbohydrates and calories tends to be easier for them to implement. Vegetarians are also naturally inclined to like lettuce, broccoli, and cauliflower and thus are well positioned to love the RBS framework.

As for adapting, as you browse through all of the recipes and take note of the few vegetarian ones, do know that all of them are completely adaptable to a vegetarian or vegan diet. Where there is meat, replace it with a meat alternative, such as tofu, tempeh, seitan, or jackfruit, or you may prefer to use the various faux meats available, such as soy chorizo, black bean burgers, and Beyond Meat products. Depending on the meat replacement item you are using, you may choose to add it in with the vegetables or add it to the top of the skillet toward the end, especially if texture is important. If you are using tofu, pat it with a paper towel to reduce the moisture and fry it a bit separately. Tofu works better at the bottom of the skillet, where it can soak up the sauce.

Replace dairy cheese with vegan cheese, which is typically made from nuts, soy, or seeds, or alternatively, simply add avocado and/or nuts to a dish. Normally, I get concerned about people adding calorie-dense items, such as avocado, nuts, and seeds, but you may end up with an awfully sparse meal without them, depending on what you are excluding from the recipe. As always, do a calorie check to make sure you are in a calorie deficit.

All of those items will have more carbs than meat, because meat is a zero-carbohydrate food. Is this a real problem? I doubt it. Would it be easier to eat meat in these meals? Apparently I think so, because that's basically why I eat meat.

TWO MEALS

Some people need to eat twice for calorie reasons or for medication reasons. Some people just feel the need to eat twice. (Some people even feel the need to eat three times, but I'll let you work that variation out on your own.)

My husband is a great example. First, his maintenance calorie level is much higher than mine. He can follow the RBS framework for weight loss and lose massive amounts of weight because he is in a deeper calorie deficit than many of us would be. He spent some weeks doing just that and learned that a better long-game approach for his 20- to 30-pound weight loss was to find a structure that could take him into maintenance. He implemented a two-meal model that looked a whole lot like this: a midmorning meal of eggs and sausage and a midafternoon RBS-inspired meal, a meal I call "RBS-lite" because it tends to be a bit smaller than my one meal.

This approach has worked extraordinarily well for him. He eats plenty but also employs the bright-line approach that I advocate. He has effectively cut out the biggest offenders in his weight gain at the same time: nighttime chips and beer.

TWO OR MORE MEALS FOR MEDICATION REASONS

When you need to take medication with food more than once a day, you will need an implementation plan. Some people simply move to a two-meal model, others move to more of a one-plus model. In a two-meal model, you would eat two smaller meals, distributing the quantity and calories across the two meals as you choose. With one-plus meals, you might choose to have one large meal and then one mini-meal of "just enough" for medication purposes. How much food is enough? This is a great question for your pharmacist in light of your own medication, but something fatty usually wins here. Fat is least likely to affect blood sugar and provides some stomach coating for the medication. Some people will eat a bit of cheese or a couple of pork rinds.

POSTBARIATRIC MULTIPLE MEALS

The smaller stomach of postbariatric patients does not allow for one of these giant meals, but the good news is that people with bariatric surgery often do not have the same level of hunger they used to have. A key strategy is to decide on your nutrition and then dole it out over four or so hours. Some people will make one of the recipes in this book, for instance, but take far longer to eat it than I would with my own ridiculously big stomach.

Whatever specific situation you find yourself in, there is very likely an adaptation that will work well for you. Do consider that your measure of success in any choice for these adaptations should be a simple one: Will this choice support your long-term goals in a way that is better than your choices of yesterday? Your only basis of comparison should be the "you" of yesterday. Look for the little tweaks to make tomorrow better.

chapter twelve

Conclusion

The meals in this book—their preparation, their ingredients—are simple, almost embarrassingly so. Do not expect me to win a big culinary award for these creations. There is simply no universe where they deserve any award for culinary mastery. However, if you find yourself out hiking on a vacation in Banff or Iceland, be sure to send me a postcard because that really is why any of us should care at all about these ridiculously simple meals.

In fact, a theme here and one you may have noticed more and more often in my messages is what I think of as "our value for food." We have struggled with our weight because we have a high value for food—for its flavors and textures, for the feeling of satisfaction it gives us when we are feeling down. That's exactly why we find ourselves rummaging in the refrigerator and freezer: we are seeking something from all of that food, but what we need is not in there at all. When we cave and then start kicking ourselves further and making it all that much worse, we find all of our emotions so completely tied up with food that it becomes difficult to extricate ourselves from it. If we stop the food rummaging and work actively to find solutions elsewhere, the value we ascribe to food flavors and sensations will change and our lives overall will become easier and more enriched.

We need to change our value for food and replace it with other values. You will see a clear example of that in a YouTube video I made with a nine-day food diary during one of my family vacations. So many of our family vacations of the past would have been focused on which restaurants we were discovering. The video shows my focus on the "not food" category. I hiked through the Rocky Mountains and nearly to the top of Zion's formidable Angel's Landing. I did all of it while eating one daily meal based on the Ridiculously Big Salad framework, right out of hotel after hotel.

On that vacation, I sought experiences and pleasures that were completely unrelated to food, and I seek to do that on a smaller scale every day, wherever I might be. Today at home as I write this book, I will take to the hillside and its fresh air and explore in some way or work on a bit of a project.

This approach gets easier over time. I have essentially practiced this way of eating every day for five years now, and I mindfully set aside any old expectations I had about "vacation eating." There may be some vacations that center on eating—and that is a story for another day, because I suspect I need to practice a bit more taking vacations that are not centered on eating. Activities such as my nine-day road trip really train the brain that life is not all about food. I reinforced that life lesson in myself on that road trip and essentially rewarded myself with a bucket-list hiking experience, an experience that in itself rewards me for having changed my own value for food.

I used this framework to lose 140 pounds (63 kilograms) and then leaned hard into it during the aftermath of the forest fire, appreciating even more the role my technocratic side played in my weight loss. I worked to keep that side of me at the helm, especially on the bad days. As we get older, it is sure easy to appreciate how critical it is to get through those bad days. It is a universal problem we share, and it is one of multiple key reasons that we find ourselves way up there on the scale.

Use the recipes in this book to take care of the business of eating. Set your intention to eat this way (or some adapted version of it) every day and especially on the bad days. Put your business self in charge, handling your eating in more of a technocratic fashion. Enjoy your food and then draw the line on your eating. Go forth and be awesome with the rest of your day. It really is as simple as that, and as I always say: it is the simplest and most difficult thing you're about to do.

P.S. Seriously! Send me a postcard!

appendix

Ingredient Guide

THE VEGETABLE FOUNDATION INGREDIENT LIST

If you figure each dish is about 12 ounces (340 grams) of the vegetable base, included is a list of the carbohydrate content of each vegetable, per 12 ounces, listed from least to most net carbohydrates. You may eat more or less. I don't feel like this decision is what got us fat, and so I leave you to decide if you're only going to eat 10 ounces or if you'll go big and eat 16 ounces.

For comparison purposes, I included potatoes and sweet potatoes at the bottom of the list. They are high in carbohydrates and calories, and I avoid them. Onions and carrots are fairly high, but you are likely not eating anywhere near 12 ounces. I often add onions for flavor. If a cabbage mix comes with the grated carrots, I eat them. In the gray area is kale, and you might decide to exclude it. I pretty much eat any of the greens and do not worry about their carbohydrate content. I do know that in my case I did not get fat on kale and consequently tend not to worry about it.

With any vegetable (as with any food), a good rule to apply is: "Will this food cause me to overeat?" While one sweet potato is not likely a big issue, a community member reported eating five in a sitting. Roasted radishes or roasted beets might have the same effect for some people. Choose a vegetable base for your meal that will help you be satisfied and walk away.

Vegetable (12 ounces [340 g])	Total Carbs	Fiber	Net Carbs	Calories
Spinach	12	7	5	78
Celery	10	5	5	50
Asparagus	13	7	6	70
Eggplant	19	12	7	80
Radish	12	5	7	54
Zucchini	11	3	8	60
Cauliflower	16	8	8	85
Collard greens	17	9	8	130
Swiss chard	15	7	8	70
Tomato	13	4	9	60
Bell pepper	16	5	11	72
Green beans	24	12	12	105
Cabbage (½ head)	25	10	15	110
Okra	24	11	15	110
Broccoli	24	9	15	115
Brussels sprouts	30	7	17	135
Carrot	32	9	23	140
Kale	36	7	29	180
Onion	34	5	29	142
Sweet potato	68	10	58	300
Potato	72	7	65	320

THE PROTEIN LIST

My rule of thumb with protein is to buy the least processed and the highest quality I can afford and just do the best I can with those goals. Recipes in this book used processed meat mainly for the convenience, but if you were to fine-tune your eating further for the health long game, you could completely level-up by cutting out the processed meats (e.g., sausage and bacon). You could purchase meats with a better fatty acid profile, in particular from animals living in the wild. These are definitely better long-game strategies. But do you know what a more fundamental long-game strategy is? Losing weight. Do not get caught up in the gourmet foodie "what to eat" discussions about wild foods at the expense of your main goal. If you don't have the money to buy higher-end protein items, buy what you can to meet your goal. Use your future svelte self to learn to hunt, and go out and harvest your own venison on your good days.

HERBS AND SPICES

Freshness is king in the world of dried herbs and spices. If you have ten-year-old spices in your cupboard, you will not get as much flavor out of them as you would from a fresher source. That said, one solution is to use more of an old herb or spice until that container is empty and then buy a new one.

Annatto. This optional spice is used in curry sauces for its red color.

Curry paste. Many curry pastes are available in Asian grocery stores and are a convenient way to whip up a quick curry dish.

OILS

Mild-tasting cooking oil. My choice in this category is avocado oil from a better-known company. The cheap bottles at the dollar store could very well be any oil at all. Those companies do not tend to keep an eye on their supply chain.

Light olive oil is an option, but a problem that both the light olive oil and avocado oil industries face is fraud: companies make more money filling up the bottle with a cheaper oil and selling it as light olive oil (or avocado oil). In the light olive oil category, there is really no good way for us consumers to know if it is actually olive oil. Fraud is rampant, and the big question, of course, is: If it is not olive oil, what is in the bottle? I do roll the dice on this sometimes and buy light olive oil in bulk at Costco. Actually, truth be told, my husband buys it, and I then use it.

The better brands in the avocado oil industry tend to monitor their supply chain a little better than others. You will notice that Chosen is starting to sell guacamole because, as a company, it is connected to actual, specific avocado trees, not just to a middleman supplier. To me that is at least a signal that we can have a bit more confidence in what is in the bottle. (If I seem ever skeptical, it is because I am ever skeptical about label claims.)

Sesame oil. You will only use a bit of this oil for flavor. It is too high in inflammatory omega-6 oils to use as a primary cooking oil. It is available at any major store. Refrigerate after opening.

SWEETENERS: STEVIA AND MONK FRUIT

My go-to sweetener is stevia. It is an extract from an herb (*Stevia rebaudiana*), one I grow in my garden. Monk fruit is an actual fruit, about the size of a small orange. Both are natural sweeteners that may not affect our blood sugar. I buy stevia powder and liquid from Trader Joe's. There are many companies that make stevia products, and they all have slightly different flavor profiles.

SEASONING BLENDS

Each of the recipes in this book has seasonings, but one task you may enjoy is to shop for seasoning blends or make some of your own. You can match a favorite seasoning blend with a vegetable base and protein and be ready to go in minutes. With commercial blends, watch for added sugar and try to reduce the number of ingredients with names you cannot pronounce.

In terms of making your own, careful readers of the digital version of this book noted a common base seasoning in each of these recipes and then whipped up a base to keep on hand. Yes, that was exactly my intention: to mention in a little sidebar such as this that you could save a step or two by mixing equal parts garlic powder, onion powder, salt, and pepper. Of course, if you do not like onion powder, you can save a step or two by mixing equal parts garlic powder, salt, and pepper.

As you shop for a sweetener to try, do look carefully at labels. There are quite a number of products on the market that would have you believe they are pure stevia or monk fruit when, in fact, they are blends, sometimes with very little stevia in them. For example, Truvia is a blend of stevia and erythritol, a sugar alcohol. Stevia in the Raw combines stevia and dextrose. Sugar alcohols may be an option for you, but they do cause intestinal distress in many people (and maybe in anyone who consumes too much of them).

Artificial sweeteners like sucralose and aspartame are controversial, and research shows they affect our blood sugar even though they are calorie-free. However, in general, the research on sweeteners is only emerging, and we really do not know for sure where we are headed. My choice is to use natural sweeteners, and I just cross my fingers that we do not learn something sinister about them in the future. That would be a sad day.

DAIRY

All of the dairy products in this book tend to be lower in carbohydrates, but it never hurts to check the label on a product that is new to you. The big caution with dairy in these recipes is not adding more than you need, calorie-wise.

APPLE CIDER VINEGAR

A number of companies sell apple cider vinegar with "the mother." The mother is the sediment at the bottom of the jar and is the culture used in making the vinegar. The sediment is healthy; swish the bottle to get some of that sediment into your salads. Definitely do not buy cider vinegar in a one-gallon plastic bottle from a warehouse store.

Other vinegars. Although apple cider vinegar is the only one I use in this book, you can use other vinegars in the recipes here, including your homemade concoctions. Just be mindful of the carb amount. Some vinegar products have a surprising amount of carbohydrates.

PANTRY ITEMS

Canned mushrooms. Always check labels, but canned mushrooms do not tend to have surprises.

Capers. This is an optional pickled condiment available in the pickled section at any major grocer.

Coconut cream. This is a richer version of coconut milk, but brands vary a great deal. Coconut milk is a reasonable substitution. It adds liquid and imparts flavor.

Mustard (Dijon, yellow). Find a mustard that you love, and you will love it in your RBS recipes as well.

Peanut powder. Peanut powder or peanut flour is a handy ingredient to have around; however, check for carbohydrates as this product does have some carbs. Try to find one without added sugar. You can use a regular peanut butter in salad dressings as well, but I like the convenience of the powder and the reduced calories. The reduced calories come from defatting the peanut butter, but peanut oil is not prized for its properties, so I like to get my fat in the rest of the salad dressing. If you go the regular peanut butter route, check for carbohydrates.

Pesto (basil). Make or buy a pesto sauce. Watch the carbohydrate content of the sauce, but you can typically find them in the 3- to 5-gram range for the approximate quarter cup you will likely use.

Salsa verde. Make or buy a basic salsa verde with no added sugar. (This is just a green salsa made with tomatillos instead of tomatoes.)

Soy sauce, tamari sauce, liquid aminos. Each of these items gives you a soy sauce flavor, though some people prefer the Japanese fermented tamari sauce, others the liquid aminos.

Tomato paste. I buy paste without added sugar. Check the label. The tomato paste in tubes can be a great option for us because it stores in the refrigerator nicely.

Acknowledgments

The production of this book survived literal wildfires, taking longer than it should have, largely because I lived some months in my own troubled little nest, lined with forest ashes. I sure hope we don't find many mistakes in this book, as a result. They are surely my own, but I'm also inclined to blame the Windy Fire.

This book would likely have taken another seventeen years without help from my husband Sander, my son Frederick, Peter Holm and his design work, and Kate Mueller's editing. Recipe help came from Anna Sul and her talented children and from Celeste McIntyre. Lots of people provided feedback on the digital version, with special hat tips to Jackie Patti, Liz Byers, Georgia Baker, and Sara Carter. It surely does take a village!

STAY CONNECTED

Over the last four years of the life of our unexpected little Eat Like a Bear! community, we have learned a whole lot about weight loss. We learn more each day. Our way of eating is highly effective, a point which cannot be missed with all our weight loss success.

However, making good eating decisions daily for the long game is a whole other kettle of fish. It is becoming increasingly clear that long-term weight maintenance is far more likely if we build support structures around ourselves — family, friends, therapists, encouraging doctors.

We each need to build structures in our lives.

As a supplement to our social networks, it is my intention to improve the support structures we offer in our digital community. As you discover this book, check out our digital offerings for our latest resources, particularly our affordable member program designed for this exact purpose.

Stay connected: EatLikeaBear.com